Case Studies in Oncology Nursing

TEXT AND REVIEW

CATHY C. FORTENBAUGH, RN, MSN, AOCN
AIM Higher Program Coordinator
Clinical Nurse Specialist
Pennsylvania Oncology Hematology Associates
Philadelphia, PA

MARGARET A. RUMMEL, RN, MHA, OCN
Oncology Nurse Manager
Pennsylvania Hospital
Philadelphia, PA

JONES AND BARTLETT PUBLISHERS
Sudbury, Massachusetts
BOSTON   TORONTO   LONDON   SINGAPORE

World Headquarters

Jones and Bartlett Publishers
40 Tall Pine Drive
Sudbury, MA 01776
978-443-5000
info@jbpub.com
www.jbpub.com

Jones and Bartlett Publishers Canada
6339 Ormindale Way
Mississauga, Ontario
L5V 1J2
CANADA

Jones and Bartlett Publishers International
Barb House, Barb Mews
London W6 7PA
UK

Jones and Bartlett's books and products are available through most bookstores and online booksellers. To contact Jones and Bartlett Publishers directly, call 800-832-0034, fax 978-443-8000, or visit our website www.jbpub.com.

Substantial discounts on bulk quantities of Jones and Bartlett's publications are available to corporations, professional associations, and other qualified organizations. For details and specific discount information, contact the special sales department at Jones and Bartlett via the above contact information or send an email to specialsales@jbpub.com.

The authors, editor, and publisher have made every effort to provide accurate information. However, they are not responsible for errors, omissions, or for any outcomes related to the use of the contents of this book and take no responsibility for the use of the products described. Treatments and side effects described in this book may not be applicable to all patients; likewise, some patients may require a dose or experience a side effect that is not described herein. The reader should confer with his or her own physician regarding specific treatments and side effects. Drugs and medical devices are discussed that may have limited availability controlled by the Food and Drug Administration (FDA) for use only in a research study or clinical trial. The drug information presented has been derived from reference sources, recently published data, and pharmaceutical research data. Research, clinical practice, and government regulations often change the accepted standard in this field. When consideration is being given to use of any drug in the clinical setting, the health care provider or reader is responsible for determining FDA status of the drug, reading the package insert, reviewing prescribing information for the most up-to-date recommendations on dose, precautions, and contraindications, and determining the appropriate usage for the product. This is especially important in the case of drugs that are new or seldom used.

Library of Congress Cataloging-in-Publication Data

Fortenbaugh, Cathy C.
   Case studies in oncology nursing : text and review / Cathy C. Fortenbaugh, Margaret A. Rummel.
      p. ; cm.
   Includes bibliographical references and index.
   ISBN-13: 978-0-7637-3455-8 (pbk. : alk. paper)
   ISBN-10: 0-7637-3455-8 (pbk. : alk. paper)
   1. Cancer—Nursing—Case studies. 2. Cancer—Nursing—Examinations, questions, etc. I. Rummel, Margaret A. II. Title.
      [DNLM: 1. Neoplasms—nursing—Case Reports. 2. Neoplasms—therapy—Case Reports. 3. Oncologic Nursing—methods—Case Reports. WY 156 F7373c 2007]
   RC266.F67 2007
      610.73'698—dc22
                         2006038973
6048

Production Credits

Executive Publisher: Christopher Davis
Production Director: Amy Rose
Production Editor: Carolyn F. Rogers
Associate Editor: Kathy Richardson
Marketing Associate: Rebecca Wasley
Manufacturing Buyer: Amy Bacus
Composition: Paw Print Media
Cover Design: Anne Spencer
Cover Image: © Glow Images/age fotostock
Printing and Binding: Malloy, Inc.
Cover Printing: Malloy, Inc.

Printed in the United States of America
10 09 08 07 06   10 9 8 7 6 5 4 3 2 1

Dedications

This book is dedicated to my husband, Peter McGrath—without his support and encouragement, the book would only have been a good idea. It is also dedicated to my children, Patrick, Sean, and Donald, to Robin and her family, and my parents, whom I cherish so much; my fellow AIM Higher Program Coordinators; my coworkers at Pennsylvania Oncology Hematology Associates and the Joan Karnell Cancer Center at Pennsylvania Hospital, Supportive Oncology Services; Peg Rummel, who helped inspire me to write; and most of all the cancer patients who inspire and humble me each day.

Cathy Fortenbaugh

This book is dedicated in loving memory of my mother, who always encouraged me to try something new and strive to be the best I can be. It is also dedicated to my friends and family, Michael, Beth, Gracie, Suzy, Christian, and Emerson, whose encouragement meant so much when the going was tough and without whom I would never have completed this project; my coworkers at Pennsylvania Hospital; my coauthor Cathy Fortenbaugh, who kept me on track; and to my patients who inspire me every day to continue to make a difference.

Margaret Rummel

Contents

Foreword

This book was conceived and developed on the inpatient oncology unit at Pennsylvania Hospital, which houses the nation's first inpatient oncology unit. The impetus for this project was simple—to train new nurses caring for oncology patients and to maintain competency in experienced oncology nurses. The authors, an advanced practice oncology nurse and an oncology nurse manager, have years of experience in working with, teaching, and mentoring new nurses. Their creative approach to the process of continuing nursing education was successful on multiple levels and this success led them to share their methods with their oncology nursing colleagues through this book.

This book provides an original and highly effective way of providing practical, useful, and interesting teaching methods and information. The nurse who is new to the field of oncology will find it easier to remember concepts provided in the case study format. For the experienced nurse, it will reinforce important concepts and clinical practice issues. For the nurse educator, the case study format provides a valuable tool for both teaching and assessment of competencies in the clinical setting. For the nurse studying for the Oncology Certification Generalist (OCN) examination, this book offers a unique approach to understanding the material and provides the reasoning for choosing the interventions necessary to achieve the most effective clinical outcomes.

It is my hope that readers will benefit from the wisdom and the years of oncology nursing experience that the authors bring to this unique and practical text.

Mary Pat Lynch, CRNP, MSN, AOCN
Oncology Nurse Practitioner and Administrator
Joan Karnell Cancer Center at Pennsylvania Hospital
Philadelphia, PA

About the Authors

Cathy C. Fortenbaugh, RN, MSN, AOCN, APN, C, is the AIM Higher program coordinator and clinical nurse specialist at Pennsylvania Oncology Hematology Associates in Philadelphia, PA. AIM Higher is a nationwide quality improvement initiative designed to improve the assessment, information, and management of chemotherapy-related symptoms. She has practiced in a wide variety of inpatient and outpatient settings, including medical oncology, surgical oncology, bone marrow transplant, and nursing education. Ms. Fortenbaugh received her BSN from Widener University in Chester, PA, and her MSN in the oncology CNS track from the University of Pennsylvania in Philadelphia, PA. She has published and presented on various topics at both the national and local levels.

Margaret A. Rummel, RN, MHA, OCN, CAN, is the inpatient oncology nurse manager at Pennsylvania Hospital in Philadelphia, PA. She has practiced in a wide variety of settings as a staff nurse and manager including medical/surgical units, medical/surgical oncology, and nursing education. Ms. Rummel received her BSN from Holy Family University in Philadelphia, PA, and her MHA from Saint Joseph's University in Philadelphia, PA. She has published and presented on various topics at both the national and local levels.

Chapter

1

Cancer and Treatment-Related Anemia Case Study

CS is a 54-year-old male who will be receiving his third course of FOLFOX 6 that consists of fluorouracil (5-FU) leucovorin (Wellcovorin, folinic acid), and oxaliplatin (Eloxatin) for colorectal cancer. He tells his nurse he has become significantly short of breath, especially on exertion, progressively over the past 10 days, and that he has not been able to maintain his usual work schedule for the past week due to severe fatigue. CS is the sole provider for his wife and 2 high-school age children. He appears very anxious about his symptoms. A hemoglobin and hematocrit reveals:

Hgb 9.3 g/dl
Hct 33%

Past medical history includes triple bypass surgery at age 50 due to severe angina, hyperlipidemia, and hypertension, which are well controlled with medication.

What is CS experiencing?

CS is experiencing chemotherapy-induced anemia. Anemia affects many patients with cancer, either because of the cancer itself or the treatments that our patients undergo, including chemotherapy, surgery, and radiation. In fact, more than half of patients with cancer are affected by anemia.[1] Many patients receiving chemotherapy experience fatigue. One recent study reported that 82.4% of patients reported fatigue at their last chemotherapy visit.[2]

What function does the hemoglobin molecule have?

Hemoglobin is a protein molecule in the red blood cell that contains iron and carries oxygen throughout the body.

What happens when hemoglobin is low?

Someone with low hemoglobin has anemia and may experience debilitating symptoms such as fatigue, shortness of breath, or chest pain. Fatigue can have a significant impact on the quality of life, such as impacting a person's ability to work or perform his usual duties, as illustrated in our case study.[1]

What is hematocrit?

Hematocrit is the percentage of red cells in the bloodstream. A low hematocrit is also an indicator of anemia.

What is a normal Hgb and Hct for a female?

A range of 12-16 g/dl is normal for a female.[3]

What is a normal Hgb and Hct for a male?

A range of 14-18 g/dl is normal for a male.[3]

Would CS be classified as having anemia?

Yes, the World Health Organization defines anemia as hemoglobin less than 13 g/dl in males and less than 12 in females. Having hemoglobin lower than these numbers can significantly impact a patient's quality of life. It is important to look at the patient and his clinical symptoms as well as the hemoglobin level.[4]

Besides fatigue, chest pain, shortness of breath, and low hemoglobin and hematocrit, what are the other signs and symptoms of anemia?

Other signs and symptoms of anemia include fatigue, dizziness, pallor, hypoxia, dyspnea, chest pain, tachycardia, anorexia, nausea, indigestion, insomnia, depression, cognitive impairment, and low hemoglobin and hematocrit.[1,4]

What interventions should be done for CS?

The most common interventions are medical management utilizing an erythropoietic agent or packed red blood cell transfusion.[5]

Why are evidence-based guidelines useful in managing symptoms?

Guidelines assist practitioners in bridging the gap between research and clinical practice. Using a guideline allows one to practice according to the best available evidence. Guidelines allow for more consistent practice; an inexperienced practitioner is able to provide care in the same manner as an experienced one.[6]

CS should receive darbepoetin alfa (Aranesp) 200 mcg after his treatment is completed.

Explain how erythropoietic agents work.

Both darbepoetin alfa and epoetin alfa (Procrit) are erythropoietic agents. Darbepoetin alfa is commonly administered as a 500 mcg dose every 3 weeks and epoetin alfa is commonly administered as a 40,000 unit dose once a week. Erythropoietin controls the production of red blood cells in the bone marrow. It is produced in the kidneys in response to hypoxia and then is transported to the bone marrow. Adequate amounts of iron, B_{12}, and folate are also necessary for red blood cell production.[1]

How are darbepoetin alfa and epoetin alfa given?

Both of these medications are given as a subcutaneous injection the same day as chemotherapy.

What baseline studies are necessary before starting darbepoetin alfa or epoetin alfa?

Draw baseline erythropoietin levels. Patients who have an endogenous erythropoietin level of less than or equal to 200 units/ml will derive the optimal response from the drug. Baseline iron studies such as serum ferritin and transferritin saturation should be obtained. Serum ferritin should be 100 mg/ml or greater and transferritin saturation should be at least 20%. Iron is replaced either as an IV infusion or orally.[7]

Explain why iron is important in the treatment of chemotherapy-related anemia.

Iron is important because iron improves response to therapy and therefore assists with red blood cell production. Even when there are enough iron stores, the patient response may be longer than expected because iron cannot be supplied fast enough to keep up with the increased demand placed on the bone marrow due to erythropoietic therapy stimulation. Inflammatory cytokines from the cancer itself may also hinder the release of stored iron.[8]

Are there any side effects of erythropoietic agents that a patient needs to be aware of?

Hypertension should be controlled before starting these drugs; seizures have been reported in chronic renal patients; thrombus formation has occurred in patients with hemoglobins greater than 12 g/dl. Additional side effects include fatigue, edema, nausea, vomiting, diarrhea, fever, and shortness of breath.[3]

What comorbidities that could cause anemia should the nurse be aware of in patients receiving chemotherapy?

Patients with a cardiac history with decompensation, cerebral vascular disease, and chronic pulmonary disease cannot tolerate a lower hemoglobin level as well as someone without these comorbidities, and they could experience more complications related to anemia. This is seen in our case study.[3]

What risk factors predispose a patient for developing chemotherapy-related anemia?

Patients receiving a myelosuppressive regimen, particularly one containing a platinum-based agent, or those who have been heavily treated with chemotherapy in the past are at the greatest risk. Other factors not related to chemotherapy include bone marrow replacement by cancer cells, current or previous radiation to the bone marrow, nutritional deficiencies, renal impairment, blood loss, and preexisting anemia. In addition, certain tumor types are associated with a higher risk of developing anemia. The most significant anemia rates occur in patients with lung cancer, gynecologic cancers, and genitourinary cancers.[1,4]

Three weeks later CS returns to the clinic still complaining of fatigue. He reports that the fatigue is now moderate and he has returned to work for a full day. He is discouraged that the fatigue is still present despite the darbepoetin alfa and that it is impacting his ability to spend time with his family. He states, "It is all I can do just to go to work." CS reports that the shortness of breath is greatly improved. He asks if the darbepoetin alfa is working.

How might CS's nurse respond to this question?

It is important to educate the patient that it may take 4-6 weeks for darbepoetin alfa to work. CS has not been receiving therapy for a long enough period of time to determine the drug's effectiveness.[7]

If CS had hemoglobin of 6.5 and immediate intervention is needed, what could his nurse do?

CS may be given packed red blood cell transfusions if it is not against his personal or religious beliefs.

Describe the risks associated with blood transfusion.

Risks include allergic reactions, febrile reactions, hemolytic reactions, bacterial contamination, volume overload, hypothermia, air emboli, transmission of viruses, and human error.[4]

What is one way to reduce the risk of CS developing a transfusion reaction?

The nurse could administer the blood with a leukocyte filter. White blood cells carry antibodies, and if they were not filtered out prior to CS receiving the blood, he is likely to develop a transfusion-related reaction.[4]

What can the nurse teach CS about fatigue?

CS will need information about energy conservation, distraction, and stress management. He can be encouraged to keep a diary. Teaching surrounding energy conservation includes:

Setting priorities; his nurse should encourage him to identify important activities
Delegation of nonpriority activities and activities that CS does not need to do himself
Scheduling activities around hours of having energy
Postponing nonessential activities
Prearranging with others to perform essential tasks that cannot be postponed
Doing one activity at a time

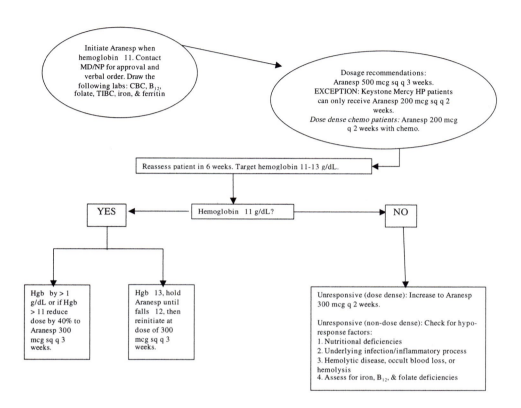

Notes: May continue Aranesp for 120 days post chemo if Hgb 13 g/dL.
HOLD DOSE IF HGB > 13 g/dL.
Discontinue therapy with resolution of symptoms of anemia.

Figure 1.1   **Aranesp Guidelines**
Source: Based on National Comprehensive Cancer Network. Clinical Practice Guidelines in Oncology v.2.2006. Cancer and Treatment-related Anemia. Available at: http://www.nccn.org/professionals/physician_gls/PDF/anemia.pdf. Accessed August 4, 2006. Also based on Aranesp Prescribing Information, 2006.

Table 1.1   **National Cancer Institute Common Toxicity Criteria: Anemia**

Toxicity	Grade				
	0	*1*	*2*	*3*	*4*
Hemoglobin (Hgb)	WNL	< LLN-10.0 g/dL	8.0- < 10.0 g/dL	6.5- < 8.0 g/dL	< 6.5 g/dL

Source: Wilkes GM, Barton-Burke M. *2005 Oncology Nursing Drug Handbook.* Sudbury, MA: Jones and Bartlett; 2005:987.

Planning ahead in the chemotherapy cycle to anticipate days of low energy and do some things in advance; e.g., meals (this is the reason for CS to keep a fatigue diary)

Scheduling naps so they will not interfere with either the daily routine or sleep

Distraction including games, music, reading, activities with friends and family, and integrative therapies such as guided imagery

Stress management activities that include relaxation exercises, humor, support groups, massage therapy, and art therapy

REFERENCES

1. Gillespie TW. Effects of cancer-related anemia on clinical and quality of life outcomes. *Clin J Oncol Nurs.* 2002;6(4):206-211.

2. Fortner BV, Moore K, Tauer K, et al. Baseline evaluation of the AIM higher initiative: patient interview data. *Support Care Cancer.* 2004;12:361-376.

3. Sabbatini P, Cella D, Chanan-Kahn A, et al. Practice guidelines in oncology: cancer and treatment related anemia. National Comprehensive Cancer Network. 2004;v.1. Available at: www.nccn.org. Accessed January 2, 2005.

4. Matthews LV. Anemia. In: Itano JK, Taoka KN, eds. *Core Curriculum for Oncology Nursing.* 4th ed. St. Louis: Elsevier Saunders. 2005;259-263.

5. Folloder J. Effects of darbepoetin alfa administered every two weeks on hemoglobin and quality of life of patients receiving chemotherapy. *Oncol Nurs Forum.* 2005;32(1): 81-91.

6. ONS evidence-based practice resource area, definitions. ONS Web site. Available at: http://onsopcontent.ons.org/toolkits/evidence/Definitions/index.shtml. Accessed June 9, 2005.

7. Chu E, DeVita V, eds. Darbepoetin alfa. *Physicians' Cancer Chemotherapy Drug Manual.* Sudbury, MA: Jones and Bartlett; 2005:118-121.

8. Henry DH. Supplemental iron: a key to optimizing the responses of cancer related anemia to rHuEPO? *Oncologist.* 1998:275-278.

2

Anxiety in the
Cancer Patient Case Study

VB is a 45-year-old female starting high-dose chemotherapy for newly diagnosed non-Hodgkin's lymphoma at an outpatient clinic. VB has no past medical history. She tells her nurse that she follows a vigorous diet and exercise routine. VB is married, has no children and is employed as an attorney at a well-known law firm in town. Her nurse is meeting VB for the first time for a pre-chemotherapy teaching session. VB states she is anxious about the upcoming treatment and is having trouble focusing on the teaching session. She gets up several times and paces around the room. She says, "I have always been in control of my life and this feels scary. I exercise, I eat right, I do all the right things and still I got cancer. What did I do wrong?" VB's husband is not present with her at this teaching session. She states "I told him not to come even though he wanted to be here because I do not want him to see me like this." She then asks about some supportive care therapies that she could participate in to help her manage the feelings she is experiencing about her diagnosis and treatment. She is specifically interested in yoga and meditation.

What is VB experiencing?

As VB herself stated she is experiencing anxiety related to diagnosis and treatment.

What is anxiety?

Anxiety is an emotional and physiologic response to a perceived threat with an increase in alertness, tension, and sympathetic nervous system response.[1] Anxiety is a common, normal response to stressful situations such as a cancer diagnosis or caring for someone with cancer.

What are the risk factors for developing anxiety in cancer patients?

Risk factors can be placed into four different categories: disease-related anxiety, treatment-related anxiety, situational anxiety, or preexisting anxiety disorders. Disease-related anxiety varies, depending where in the cancer trajectory the patient is. When patients are first diagnosed with cancer or when there is a real or perceived change in their condition, they may feel nervous, afraid, and overwhelmed. The uncertainty of prognosis is a factor. Inadequate symptom control at any phase of a patient's illness can cause anxiety. Anxiety is often found along with dyspnea, pain, anticipation of pain, fatigue, weakness, nausea, urinary retention, constipation, and insomnia.[2] Treating the anxiety alone cannot achieve adequate overall symptom control. Cancer itself can be a contributing factor. Hormone-secreting tumors are directly responsible for creating anxiety, as are brain metastases in areas that affect physical comfort, breathing, or circulation. Abnormal metabolic states such as hypoxia, pulmonary embolism, delirium, sepsis, bleeding, and hypoglycemia all contribute to the presence of anxiety in a cancer patient.[3] The patient with advanced cancer may be experiencing anxiety not because of a fear of death but because of real or perceived issues of uncontrolled pain or other symptoms, isolation, abandonment, and dependency.[4] Treatment-related anxiety is complex. Prolonged treatment, intense treatment, or hospitalization can contribute to anxiety. Medications that can cause anxiety include corticosteroids, neuroleptics, tyroxine, bronchodilators, antihistamines, decongestants, beta-adrenergic stimulants, and opioids. A change in the goal of treatment can be anxiety producing.[3] Some situational anxiety is created when the patient experiences role-related changes and losses such as health, status, finances, family roles and relationships, and social interactions. The patient may not have access to activities that she formerly enjoyed that provided stress relief. Excessive nicotine or caffeine can cause anxiety. Withdrawal from addictive substances can cause anxiety as well. Some examples of preexisting anxiety disorders include generalized anxiety, phobias, panic attacks, and posttraumatic stress.[3-4]

How common is anxiety in cancer patients?

According to one study, 44% of patients with cancer reported some anxiety and 23% reported significant anxiety.[4]

What are some common emotional signs and symptoms of anxiety?

Some common emotional signs and symptoms of anxiety include verbalization of feeling anxious, irritability, crying easily, self-doubt, and self-blame.[3]

What are some cognitive signs and symptoms of anxiety?

Some cognitive signs and symptoms of anxiety include difficulty concentrating, difficulty with memory, difficulty making decisions, and disorientation.[3]

What are some physical signs and symptoms of anxiety?

Some common signs and symptoms of anxiety include decreased hearing or visual acuity, feelings of heaviness, flushing, sweating, pacing, increased muscle tension, trembling, shaking, dizziness, irritability, sweating, fatigue, insomnia, changes in sleep, headaches, shortness of breath, rapid or irregular heartbeat, dry mouth, diarrhea, weight loss or weight gain, and frequent urination.[3]

Why is it important to address anxiety in cancer patients?

Anxiety can be a normal part of adapting to a cancer diagnosis. Most patients and families experience anxiety during the diagnostic period. If anxiety is untreated it can significantly affect quality of life.[4]

How is anxiety treated?

Determining the cause of anxiety is the first step because it will help determine the best management approach. VB's nurse should provide a calm environment and listen in a sensitive manner. She should help the patient identify feelings such as vulnerability, hopelessness, helplessness, fear, loss of control, and fear of the unknown. She can refer VB to the appropriate counseling and/or a support group. She should promptly address any unrelieved symptoms. If the cause is medication induced, her nurse should contact the provider to stop or reduce the medication if possible and monitor for resolution of anxiety. If the symptoms are due to opioid or benzodiazepine withdrawals, the ideal situation is dose reduction of 25% every 1-3 days. If the cause is alcohol withdrawal, a long-acting benzodiazepine may reduce the withdrawal symptoms and anxiety. If the anxiety is due to caffeine withdrawal, the nurse should encourage VB to gradually decrease the amount of caffeine intake. If the anxiety is from nicotine withdrawal, she should encourage the use of the nicotine patch, gum, or inhaler to reduce cravings. If encephalopathy is a factor, an appropriate workup may be indicated. Radiation therapy and corticosteroids are used to treat brain metastasis. She should address the patient's concerns regarding spiritual issues, refer as necessary for spiritual counseling, and support prayer and meditation. She should assist the patient in maintaining her spiritual connections. Behavioral methods to help treat anxiety include relaxation techniques, music therapy, guided imagery, visualization, art therapy, music therapy, self-hypnosis, humor, massage, and exercise. Cognitive therapies include biofeedback, distraction, education, meditation, and reframing the situation.[2] **Table 2.1** summarizes anxiolytic agents that are useful for short-term symptomatic treatment.

Table 2.1   **Anxiolytic Agents for Short-Term Symptomatic Treatment**

Class	Medication	Discussion
Nonbenzodiazepines	Buspirone (Buspar)	Less potential for sedation or abuse. Optimal therapeutic benefit after 3-4 weeks. Must be taken regularly. Maximum daily dose 60 mg/day divided into 3 doses.
Antihistamines	Hydroxyzine (Atarax) Diphenhydramine (Benadryl)	Not recommended in geriatric patients because of cholinergic effects.
Benzodiazepines	Short-acting lorazepam (Ativan) Oxazepam (Serax)	Addictive, have withdrawal potential. Potentiate opioid effects.

Source: Adapted from Vogel WH, Wilson MA, Melvin MS, eds. Anxiety. *Advanced Practice Palliative Care Guidelines.* 2004; Philadelphia, PA: Lippincott, Williams, and Wilkins; 2004:310-317.

How is VB's anxiety going to affect the teaching session that has been planned for her?

Some level of anxiety is helpful to patients during stressful situations. Mild anxiety can help patients become more alert to their environment. As attention and awareness are stimulated, concentration sharpens. However, if anxiety becomes moderate to severe, concentration is negatively affected. VB will have difficulty retaining information because her anxiety is not at a mild level. It will negatively affect her ability to learn. This, in turn, can have an impact on her ability to manage chemotherapy-related symptoms. It could have serious consequences for symptoms such as neutropenia. VB's anxiety needs to be managed before any teaching can take place.[5]

Describe how the nurse should specifically intervene for VB.

VB should be encouraged to meet with the oncology social worker and psychologist at the clinic and referred to an appropriate support group. She can also be given information about how she can gain access to the 2 complementary and alternative medicine (integrative) therapies that she is interested in, yoga and meditation.

What is complementary and alternative medicine?

Complementary and alternative medicine (CAM) is a group of diverse medical and healthcare systems, practices, and products that are not considered to be part of conventional medicine.[6]

What is the difference between complementary and alternative medicine?

The 2 terms are very different from one another according to the National Center for Complementary and Alternative Medicine (NCCAM) at the National Institutes of Health. Complementary medicine is used together along with conventional medicine. Alternative medicine is used in place of conventional medicine. One example of a complementary medicine is acupuncture used along with gabapentin (Neurontin) to treat neuropathic pain. One example of an alternative therapy is utilizing a special diet to treat breast cancer instead of the recommended surgery, chemotherapy, and radiation.[6]

What is integrative medicine?

The NCCAM defines integrative medicine as the practice of combining mainstream medical therapies and complementary and alternative therapies for which there is good scientific evidence of safety and efficacy.[6]

Is the use of complementary and alternative therapies common in the United States?

Yes, according to a survey released in May 2004 by NCCAM, 36% of adults use some form of complementary or alternative therapy. These therapies include acupuncture, meditation, and herbal supplements. When prayer is used for health reasons, the number increases to 62%. Interestingly, many of these patients do not report their practices to their health care providers.[7]

Does VB fit the profile of someone who is most likely to use CAM?

Yes, the NCCAM survey reported that predictors of CAM among patients with cancer include being female, better educated, in higher socioeconomic status, and younger than those who do not use CAM.[6]

Table 2.2   **5 Categories of CAM**

Type	Description	Examples
1. Alternative medical systems	Built upon complete systems of theory and practice, these systems have evolved apart from and earlier than the conventional medical approach.	Homeopathic medicine, naturopathic medicine, traditional Chinese medicine, and ayurveda.
2. Mind–body interventions	Used to enhance the mind's capacity to affect body functions and symptoms.	Cognitive-behavioral therapy, support groups, meditation, prayer, mental healing and art, music, or dance therapy.
3. Biologically based therapies	Use of substances found in nature such as herbs, foods, and vitamins.	Aloe vera for burns, ginger for nausea, and chamomile tea for sleep.
4. Manipulative and body-based methods	Based on manipulation and/or movement of one or more parts of the body.	Shiatsu massage and chiropractic manipulation.
5. Energy therapies	Use of energy fields.	Qi gong, Reiki, therapeutic touch, magnetic fields.

Source: Based on Get the facts: what is complementary and alternative medicine? Available at http://nccam.nih.gov/health/whatiscam/. Accessed April 24, 2006.

Why is it important for nurses caring for people with cancer to have competency related to CAM?

Oncology nurses care for the whole person. It is important to assess the cultural, psychological, and spiritual components that affect the patients, cancer care preferences, and choices. Knowledge provides the nurse with the opportunity to discuss issues important to cancer patients and continue to maintain patient safety.[6]

What are the 5 major types of CAM?

The NCCAM classifies CAM into 5 major categories: alternative medical systems, mind–body interventions, biologically based therapies, manipulative and body based methods, and energy therapies (**see Table 2.2**).[6]

REFERENCES

1. Holland J, Boettger J. Depression and anxiety. In: Berger A, ed. *Handbook of Supportive Care in Oncology*. New York: CMP Healthcare Media, Oncology Publishing Group; 2005:169-194.

2. Vogel WH, Wilson MA, Melvin MS. Anxiety. *Advanced Practice Oncology Palliative Care Guidelines*. Philadelphia, PA: Lippincott Williams and Wilkins; 2004:310-317.

3. Brant JB. Coping: psychological issues. In: Itano JK, Taoka KN, eds. *Core Curriculum for Oncology Nursing*. 4th ed. St. Louis, MO: Elsevier Saunders; 2005:32-33.

4. National Cancer Institute. Anxiety disorder. Available at: http://www.cancer.gov/cancertopics/pdq/supportivecare/anxiety/healthprofessional. Accessed July 30, 2006.

5. Stephenson PL. Before the teaching begins: managing patient anxiety prior to providing education. *Clin J Oncol Nurs*. 2006;10(2):241-245.

6. NCCAM. Get the facts: what is complementary and alternative medicine? Available at: http://nccam.nih.gov/health/whatiscam. Accessed March 31, 2006.

7. Arias D. Alternative medicine's popularity prompts concern: use of alternative and complementary remedies on the rise. Medscape Web site. Available at: http://www.medscape.com/viewarticle/484309. Accessed March 30, 2006.

3

Brachytherapy Case Study

JS is a 53-year-old female diagnosed with stage IV cervical cancer being admitted to the oncology unit for brachytherapy. She will be in the unit for 3 days. The nurse assigns her to the room that is specified for patients receiving brachytherapy on that floor.

What is brachytherapy?

Brachytherapy is the treatment of cancers with radioactive sources placed either temporarily or permanently into the tumor, next to a tumor, or into a lumen. The advantage of brachytherapy is the ability of delivering high doses of radiation to the tumor while sparing the surrounding tissue. Low-dose radiation (as in this case) is delivered over a period of a few days and high-dose radiation is delivered over a few minutes. The radioactive material is sealed in a container and never comes in direct contact with the patient.[1-2] JS will go to the operating room and have an applicator (sealed container) placed. The radiation oncologist and radiation physicist will load the radioactive source into the applicator in the patient's room.

What type of preparation should JS's nurse have received?

Those caring for JS should have attended a radiation safety class, where they learned the essential concepts of time, distance, and shielding. They are required to update this class yearly and their supervisor may monitor their competency yearly.[1]

What do the concepts of time, distance, and shielding mean?

The concept of time means that caregivers will minimize the amount of time spent near radioactive sources. Staff is expected to work quickly and efficiently. The same caregiver should not be assigned to the patient for the duration of her stay. Caregiving should be rotated.[1-2]

The concept of distance means that the intensity of radiation decreases as the distance increases. Staff should be as far away from radioactive sources as possible.[1-2]

The concept of shielding means that a shield is placed around the patient to decrease the exposure to caregivers. The type of shielding and the thickness depend on the type and energy of the radioactive source.[1-2] JS will have portable lead shields placed at the sides and foot of the bed.

What type of preparation did or will JS receive? What plans are made for her stay, and what preparations are done to her room?

JS had extensive teaching prior to admission. She is comfortable that staff will limit the time they spend in her room. She also knows that everything that enters the room will stay in the room until cleared by the radiation physicist. Meals will come on disposable trays. The staff will try to multitask while in the room rather than make multiple visits. She is aware that there will be very minimal bathing and linen changes. She brought music, books on tape, and other activities with her to provide distraction. Children and pregnant women (visitors and staff) are unable to enter the room during the admission. The radiation physicist will draw a line in the room that marks where visitors should stand or sit. The radiation physicist will determine how much time visitors can spend in the room. A Foley catheter will be inserted and remain for the duration of the hospitalization. After the applicator is placed, JS will have vaginal packing placed around it to help hold it in place. JS is on a low-residue diet and is instructed about the diet prior to admission. She will also receive a medication such as loperamide (Imodium) to help assure that she does not have a bowel movement. JS understands that she should report the urge to have a bowel movement. After the applicator is placed in the operating room, the patient will only have the head of the bed raised to 15 degrees. If any turning in bed is necessary, she will be logrolled from side to side.[1-2]

The patient asks what the difference is between chemotherapy and brachytherapy. How should the nurse respond?

Chemotherapy is a systemic treatment and brachytherapy is a form of radiation therapy that is used for local treatment of JS's cervical cancer.

Where are radiation warning signs and instructions placed?

Warning signs are placed on the patient's door, on the chart, and on the patient armband. Necessary instructions about the source and exposure rate, as well as specific instructions for nurses and visitors, such as length of time allowed in the room, is placed on the chart.[1-2]

How is the level of exposure to the radioactive source monitored?

Anyone who works with patients receiving brachytherapy must put on a film badge or dosimeter prior to entering the room. The film badge contains small photographic film, and the dosimeter monitors radiation through a thin layer of aluminum oxide.[1]

Where should the nurses wear their film badges?

They should wear them on the trunk of their bodies. This is where their vital organs are located.[1]

A nurse is going to lunch. The coworker who will be covering for her asks to borrow her film badge. What should the nurse heading to lunch tell her?

Anyone working with brachytherapy should never wear someone else's badge since the purpose of the badge is to measure how much exposure each person has received.[1] If the substitute does not have her own film badge, she cannot care for the patient. Anyone going to lunch must arrange for someone who has a film badge to cover for her.

A nurse enters a room and notices what might be a radioactive source on the bed. What should she do next?

She must never touch a radioactive source. She should call the radiation safety officer, who uses a long-handled, tonglike forceps to pick up the source (**Figure 3.1**). The source is placed in a lead-lined container called a "pig."[1-2]

How is the room cleared as "safe" after brachytherapy is finished and the radioactive source is removed?

A Geiger counter is used to survey the room, the patient, trash, linen, and anything else in the room before it is considered clear for general use.[1-2]

What should the nurse do if JS unexpectedly respiratory arrested?

The nurses should proceed with their usual CPR procedures, trying to stay behind the lead shield. If this proceeds into a code situation, all staff should be wearing their film badges. If the code is anticipated to be lengthy, staff should rotate in and out of the room until the radioactive source is removed. The radiation safety

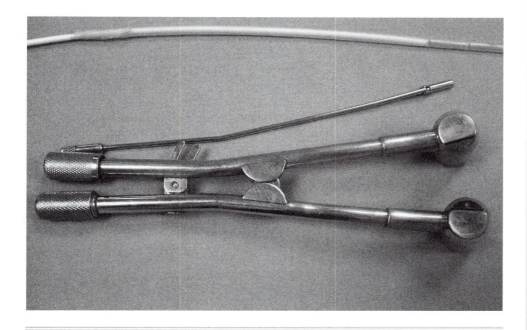

Figure 3.1   **Fletcher-style applicator.**

officer should be emergently called to remove the radioactive source. This must be done before JS is transported. JS must be logrolled to place the backboard behind her since the head of her bed cannot be raised more than 15 degrees for this type of brachytherapy.[1-2]

What factors go into determining what room is used for brachytherapy on the floor?

Potential for exposure for individuals in the room surrounding the brachytherapy room as well as rooms above and below it must be considered. Many rooms are placed next to a stairwell in an area with little activity on the floors above and below it. The radiation physicist will determine which rooms can safely house brachytherapy patients.[1-2]

REFERENCES

1. Witt ME. Nursing implications of radiation therapy. In: Itano JK, Taoka KN, eds. *Core Curriculum for Oncology Nursing*. 4th ed. St. Louis, MO: Elsevier Saunders; 2005:748-762.

2. Behrend SW. Radiation therapy treatment planning. In: Yarbro CH, Frogge MH, Goodman M, Groenwald S, eds. *Cancer Nursing Principles and Practice*. 5th ed. Sudbury, MA: Jones and Bartlett; 2000:100-322.

4

Breast Cancer Case Study

RF is a 64-year-old married woman. She has 6 children, 4 of whom are female, ranging in age from 24-42. She presents to her primary physician because she found a lump in her left breast during breast self-exam. Her first child was born when she was age 22. There is a family history of breast cancer; her grandmother was diagnosed at age 50 and her aunt at age 60. She has 2 sisters, both of whom have breast cancer and were diagnosed in their 40s. Her mother died when she was 88 years old and did not have a history of cancer. RF related that she started menstruating at age 12 and reached menopause naturally around age 55. She is 5 feet 7 inches tall and weighs 150 pounds.

What risk factors does RF have related to a possible breast cancer diagnosis?

RF has several risk factors. First, she is female with a strong family history of breast cancer, including her grandmother, aunt, and 2 first-degree relatives who are her sisters, both of whom were diagnosed at an early age. She is 64 years old, and breast cancer incidence increases with age. RF had an early menarche and menopause occurred rather late at age 55. Both of these are risk factors for RF as this has caused her increased exposure to estrogen during her reproductive lifetime.[1-2]

Even though RF can feel a lump in her breast, her primary care physician orders a mammogram. It reveals a 5.5 cm tumor in the left upper quadrant of her breast. RF's primary care physician then refers her to a surgical oncologist. Since the breast lump is palpable, a core biopsy is done in the surgical oncologist's office. Two days later the biopsy comes back positive for invasive ductal breast cancer and she is scheduled for lumpectomy and sentinel lymph node sampling after much discussion with her surgeon and family.

What preprocedure teaching should this patient receive?

The procedure, including pre- and postprocedure care, should be explained. RF must have nothing by mouth from midnight prior to surgery. It will be performed in the surgical suite under general anesthesia. RF will need to have a support person with her to provide transportation home since she will be having same-day surgery. She needs specific instructions about where to report the morning of the surgery and what time to arrive. The procedure should be explained to RF. Her lumpectomy will be done first. It involves removal of the tumor and a margin of normal tissue surrounding it. If the tumor were nonpalpable, a needle localization procedure would be done first. This is done under ultrasound or mammography guidance. The tumor is located and a thin guide wire is placed into it to guide the surgeon. The sentinel node biopsy is done to determine if there is spread of the tumor to the axillary lymph nodes on the side of the tumor. If so, the cancer will be detected in the first lymph node to receive drainage from the tumor. This node is known as the sentinel lymph node. If it is negative then no more lymph nodes need to be removed and RF is spared an axillary dissection. The accuracy rate of sentinel node biopsies is 97.5%.[3] If the sentinel node biopsy is positive, then an axillary node dissection needs to be done in order to stage the tumor properly. If RF has signed consent for the procedure, the axillary node dissection can be done at the same time; if not, it is done at a subsequent date.[2] A blue dye and radioactive tracer are injected around the tumor bed in order to properly identify and biopsy the sentinel node. RF's nurse should explain to RF that the blue dye will turn her urine green for up to a day after the procedure. RF should be assessed for allergies to the dye or radioactive tracer. She should also explain to RF that she will have dressings in place on both the lumpectomy and sentinel node biopsy sites that she should keep on for 3 days and then remove and leave open to air. She will have steri-strips and sutures in place. The sutures will be removed in approximately 1 week at the postoperative visit. She is given a prescription for oxycodone with acetaminophen (Percocet) 5/325 and instructed to take 2 tablets every 4 hours as needed for pain. She is also instructed to report a temperature greater than 101°F or any unusual bleeding. Each surgeon's postoperative instructions may be slightly different.[2]

RF's sentinel node biopsy is positive. The surgical oncologist orders a bone scan and chest X-ray as part of the staging workup.

Why are these tests ordered for RF?

Since there was a positive sentinel node biopsy, a metastatic workup is done as part of the staging process. The chest X-ray was ordered to make sure that the cancer has not spread to the lung. The bone scan was ordered to check for metastasis to the bone. Breast cancer has an affinity to spread to the lungs and bones. In fact, bone is the most common site of metastasis. If metastasis has occurred, RF will be presented with different treatment options.[2]

RF asks about the bone scan. What should she be told?

A bone scan is done in the nuclear medicine department. A small dose of radioactive substance is injected into the vein. Other than a small needle stick, the procedure is painless. The radioactive substance will collect in the area of any bone metastasis and show up on the X-ray.

RF decides to have intraoperative radiation therapy and axillary lymph node dissection because of the positive sentinel node biopsy. She meets with the radiation oncologist.

What preoperative teaching should be done regarding these procedures?

The usual preoperative teaching should be provided for RF. This includes instructing her that she may not have anything to eat or drink after midnight prior to surgery, what time and where to report for surgery, and what she will experience postoperatively. RF will have an intraoperative radiation treatment called MammoSite. She will also have an axillary dissection due to her previous positive sentinel node biopsy. Axillary dissection involves removal of the lymph nodes on the affected side. She will be hospitalized overnight after the procedure and discharged the following day. A surgical drain, most likely a Jackson Pratt drain, will be present for about a week or until output is less than 30 ml in a 24-hour period. RF will learn how to empty the drain and measure the output. She will again be given a prescription for oxycodone and acetaminophen 5/325 every 4 hours as needed for pain. She is again instructed to call her surgeon for a fever greater than 101°F, any unusual bleeding, or any problem with the drain. Once again, individual surgeon's instructions may vary slightly.[2] MammoSite is a new operative procedure that delivers targeted radiation therapy to the tumor bed, therefore limiting damage to healthy breast tissue and decreasing the length of treatment needed.[4] The MammoSite Radiation Safety System (RTS) internally delivers radiation directly to the tissue surrounding the original tumor, minimizing radiation exposure to the rest of the breast, skin, ribs, lungs, and heart. During the lumpectomy procedure or shortly thereafter, the deflated MammoSite balloon is placed inside the tumor resection cavity. The applicator shaft, a tube connected to the balloon, remains outside the breast. Once in place, the balloon is inflated with saline to fill the cavity, the catheter site is dressed, and the patient may go home. The balloon remains inflated for the entire time that the patient is receiving radiation therapy. The patient returns to the hospital for treatment on an outpatient basis where a radioactive "seed" is inserted within the inflated balloon, beginning a 1- to 5-day sequence of treatments. No source of radiation remains in the patient's body between treatments or after the final procedure. When the therapy is concluded, the balloon is deflated and the MammoSite RTS catheter is easily removed. RF should be instructed about pain control, diet, activity, incision care, drains, the MammoSite catheter (**Figure 4.1**), and respiratory protocols

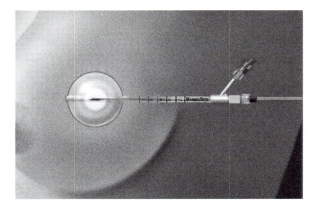

Figure 4.1   **MammoSite catheter.**
    Source: MammoSite catheter provided courtesy of Cytyc Corporation and affiliates.

after surgery, including incentive spirometry and coughing, turning, and deep breathing. While teaching RF, her nurse should assess her emotional status and coping skills, as this will have an impact on her ability to retain information.[2]

RF asks about survival rates compared to a modified radical mastectomy. What should she be told?

The long-term survival rates and reoccurrence rates are comparable between lumpectomy and axillary dissection with radiation (also known as breast-conserving surgery) and modified radical mastectomy. The breast-conservation surgery is easier to adjust to after surgery and is less disfiguring. However, mastectomy involves removal of the entire breast tissue and axillary lymph nodes so that local control with radiation is not necessary. The choice is a very personal one.[2]

What postoperative care should this patient receive?

RF's vital signs should be monitored per hospital policy and procedure for post-op patients. Vital signs generally are monitored every 4 hours for the first 24 hours. Her pain should be assessed at least every 4 hours using the 0-10 pain scale and documented accordingly. Prn pain medications should be administered as ordered if RF is experiencing any pain; relief should be assessed 30 minutes after an oral pain medication and 10 minutes after an IV pain medication. RF needs to be out of bed her first post-op night and be ambulated as soon as possible to prevent postoperative complications such as pneumonia and deep vein thrombosis. She must be encouraged to cough, turn, and deep breathe frequently and use her incentive spirometer 10 times an hour. Her incision must be assessed and her Jackson Pratt drain monitored for output. The affected arm should be elevated with the hand higher than the elbow and the elbow higher than the shoulder to facilitate lymph drainage. Intake and output are to be monitored every 4 hours. She should void within 8 hours of surgery. RF will probably be discharged the next day. Limited arm exercises such as squeezing a ball are done the first day. She should receive a physical therapy consultation prior to discharge to review arm exercises with her in order to prevent lymphedema. The arm exercises (see **Figure 4.2**) usually begin the second or third day. RF's nurse should encourage her to use the affected arm as much as possible for activities of daily living. A consultation to physical therapy for further work is necessary if full range of motion is not restored within 4-8 weeks. RF needs a social work consultation for home care if she is going home with her drains. Also, drain care, hand and arm care, and when follow-up appointments should occur are reviewed. Written materials reinforce verbal teaching.[2]

RF's surgical oncologist meets with her and informs her that the pathology report reveals stage IIIA disease with positive sentinel lymph node biopsy. Stage IIIA breast cancer has a tumor diameter greater than 5 cm with positive nodal involvement on the same side as the tumor. Metastasis has not occurred at this point.[5] She is referred to a medical oncologist to discuss further treatment.

How is breast cancer staged?

It is staged using the TNM system. T stands for tumor size, N stands for lymph node involvement, and M stands for distant metastasis. The stage of the cancer corresponds to increasing tumor involvement. The higher the stage, the more involvement is noted.

Patient Information

PENNSYLVANIA HOSPITAL
SECTION OF PHYSICAL MEDICINE AND REHABILITATION
PHYSICAL THERAPY SERVICES

POST BREAST SURGERY EXERCISES

Guidelines: Perform exercises slowly. Perform 6–8 repetitions, 3–4 times a day.

Precautions: Do not pull beyond the incisional pain. If there is drainage from the incision or the incision opens, notify your surgeon. You can relieve some chest wall tightness with gentle massage.

DAY #1 AFTER SURGERY:

1. Squeeze a sponge or rolled rag.

2. Bend and straighten your affected elbow.

3. Move your hand from "face-down" position to "face- up" position.

4. Shrug your shoulders.

5. Take a slow, deep breath through your nose. Let your chest expand. Exhale through pursed lips. Let your chest and shoulders relax.

DAY #2 AFTER SURGERY:

1. Continue to perform Day 1 exercises.
2. Touch the opposite shoulder.
3. Touch the opposite knee.
4. Comb your hair with your affected arm.
5. Reach for the small of your back with your affected arm.

Figure 4.2   **Pennsylvania Hospital hand and arm exercises.**

DAY #3 AFTER SURGERY:

1. Continue to perform Day #1 and Day #2 exercises.

2. Pendulum: standing at a table, lean forward at the waist. Allow your arm to hang loosely.

   a. Swing your arm left to right.

   b. Swing your arm forward to backward.

   c. Swing your arm in circles—both directions.

3. Wall climbing:

   a. Stand facing the wall. Slowly walk your hand up the wall until your hand is at a right angle to your body. Slowly walk your hand down the wall.

   b. Stand with your affected arm near the wall. Slowly walk your hand up the wall until your hand is at a right angle to your body. Slowly walk your hand down the wall.

DAY #12 and on:

(The following exercises should be done after drains are discharged)

These exercises should be performed twice daily for 8 repetitions.

Hold each stretch for 10 seconds.

1. Cane flexion: Lie on your back with a cane or stick in both hands. As you breathe in, slowly lift the cane up to the ceiling until your elbows are straight. As you exhale, allow arms to fall back. Pull cane back up and down towards chest.

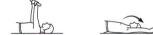

2. Cane abduction: Lie on back, holding stick as shown, with your affected arm out to the side. Using the stick for assistance, stretch your arm out to the side and overhead. Relax your arm to the side.

3. Internal rotation: Reach behind your back as shown with your affected arm. Using your other arm, grab your affected arm and pull upward.

4. External rotation: Reach up behind your head as shown. Press elbows backward so you can feel a stretch.

Figure 4.2   **Pennsylvania Hospital hand and arm exercises. (*continued*)**

What 3 nursing diagnoses are the most important for this patient?

Knowledge deficit related to her diagnosis and impending course of treatment are most important. RF has a lot to learn regarding her disease process and treatment such as chemotherapy and radiation therapy. Alteration in body image related to surgery as treatment are also important. RF will be dealing with other body image changes related to her chemotherapy and radiation therapy. She will also have impaired mobility related to her surgery, drains, and pain at the operative sites.

The pathology report reveals that she is estrogen/progesterone (ER/PR) positive, which means that her tumor is hormonally sensitive, and that she had 5 out of 13 positive lymph nodes.

After RF heals, she is referred to a medical oncologist. What type of treatment would likely be recommended for her?

Based on RF's pathology report, both chemotherapy and hormonal therapy are recommended. She already received local radiation therapy in the operating room. If she had not received the radiation in the operating room she would have received 6 weeks of radiation.

RF sees her medical oncologist for her follow-up visit. They discuss her course of treatment; her physician recommends that she receive 4 cycles of doxorubicin (Adriamycin) and cyclophosphamide (Cytoxan) followed by 4 cycles of paclitaxel (Taxol).

An oral aromatase inhibitor, anastrozole (Arimidex) is also ordered due to RF's positive ER/PR status.

Doxorubicin is a chemotherapeutic agent that acts by binding to cellular DNA and stopping its synthesis, therefore killing cancer cells. The major toxicities of this drug include myelosuppression, alopecia, nausea, vomiting, and mucositis. Sucking on ice during administration may decrease the severity of mucositis. Doxorubicin also causes cardiotoxicity. Patients should have a multiple gated acquisition (MUGA) scan prior to the start of treatment to assess a baseline cardiac status. The nurse should teach RF about measures to reduce infection such as adequate hand washing, avoiding crowds, and maintaining skin integrity. There is a maximum dose limit for this drug of 550 mg/m^2, as at higher doses there is an increased risk of cardiotoxicity. If a patient is receiving concurrent radiation therapy or has received radiation therapy, then the cumulative dose of doxorubicin is lower. Doxorubicin is a vesicant. If it extravasates, tissue damage and necrosis will occur. This drug must be administered via IV push through the side arm of a free-flowing IV, and blood return must be checked before administering it.[6]

Cyclophosphamide is a chemotherapeutic agent that interferes with DNA replication. The major toxicities of cyclophosphamide are myelosuppression, hemorrhagic cystitis, alopecia, and nausea and vomiting. Nurses should premedicate with antiemetics such as a serotonin antagonist and a steroid. RF should be taught to maintain adequate hydration of about 2-3 liters of fluid a day just after receiving cyclophosphamide to prevent hemorrhagic cystitis. She should also be advised to report burning on urination or pink or blood-tinged urine immediately, since these could be early signs that a problem is occurring. She should report a fever greater than 101°F, chills, cough, sore throat, or any other signs and symptoms of infection. RF should report any unusual bruising or bleeding and take additional measures to avoid injury. She should avoid grapefruit juice because a food-drug interaction can occur. Patients receiving concurrent radiation therapy may need a dose reduction due to additional risk of bone marrow suppression.[6]

Paclitaxel is a chemotherapeutic agent that stabilizes microtubules and inhibits cell division. It is cell-cycle specific and works in the G2 and M phases. The major toxicities include myelosuppression, alopecia, peripheral neuropathy, hypersensitivity reaction, facial flushing, myalgia, fatigue, cardiac arrhythmias, mucositis, and diarrhea. Pretreatment 30-60 minutes prior to administration of paclitaxel is necessary to prevent hypersensitivity reactions including anaphylaxis with cimetadine (Tagamet) 300 mg IV or other histamine 2 blocker, diphenhydramine (Benadryl) 50 mg IV, and dexamethasone (Decadron) 20 mg IV. PVC tubing or bags should be avoided. A 0.2-micron filter is required. RF must learn measures to prevent infection and to report infection or bleeding as outlined previously. About 45% of patients receiving paclitaxel develop peripheral neuropathy. See Case Study 15, Peripheral Neuropathy, for further information.[7]

Anastrazole is an endocrine therapy that prevents the conversion of adrenal and ovarian androgens to estrogen by inhibiting the aromatase enzyme. It interferes with proteins in all phases of the cell cycle. It is an oral agent used as adjuvant therapy in postmenopausal women who have had positive ER/PR receptors. Side effects include diarrhea, asthenia, nausea, headache, hot flashes, back pain, and peripheral edema.[7]

RF is having trouble coping with her diagnosis and treatment. What supportive services could be recommended for her and her family?

Initially, a referral to the American Cancer Society's Reach to Recovery program will put RF in contact with another woman who has had a similar surgical experience to what she had. RF can be provided with the contacts for social work, psychological counseling, physical therapy, occupational therapy, support groups, and nutritional counseling as available at the facility where she is. She should be given a list of the community resources for breast cancer patients, such as the American Cancer Society, Living Beyond Breast Cancer, The Wellness Community, and The Susan G. Komen Foundation. There are many more resources available, and these may be different for other patients, depending upon the communities where they live. If RF has computer access, she can connect to online communities related to breast cancer with a list of reliable web sites.

RF completes her course of treatment with few side effects and asks what follow-up she should have. What might some recommendations be?

The recommended follow-up includes a visit with her physician every 3 months the first year. This is usually every 6 months for the second year and then yearly after that. She will follow up with the medical oncologist for the long term since she had 5 positive axillary lymph nodes; this is considered systemic disease. She should be taught to continue breast self-exam in both her operative and unaffected breast on the same day each month since she is postmenopausal. She should continue to get her yearly mammograms and clinical breast exams on a regular basis as recommended by her physicians.[1]

What long-term issues might RF have to deal with?

RF may have to deal with many of the long-term issues faced by many cancer patients. These may include survivor guilt, fear of recurrence, lymphedema, anxiety, depression, altered body image, fear of intimacy, and change in family and social relationships. Treatment for these issues will be individual and based upon a thorough nursing assessment and the impact these issues have on RF's quality of life.

Should someone recommend genetic counseling and possible testing for RF? What about her daughters?

Yes. Due to her multiple risk factors, she should consider undergoing genetic counseling and possible testing. The genetic counselor will draw a family pedigree, look at the patient's risk factors and determine if genetic counseling is recommended. The decision to have genetic testing is a very personal one. If RF does decide to have testing, it will be for the presence of breast cancer (BRCA 1 and 2) gene mutations. These mutations are only found in 5%-10% of all breast cancers. If RF decides to test and is negative for the BRCA 1 and 2 gene mutations, then her daughters will not need to be tested. If she tests positive, her daughters might want to consider undergoing genetic counseling and possible testing. If they do not wish to have testing, they should receive follow-up appropriate for high-risk individuals. Once a specific gene mutation has been identified in a family, the genetic testing is both less expensive and easier to perform.[2,8]

RF undergoes genetic testing and is negative for the BRCA 1 and 2 gene mutations.

REFERENCES

1. American Cancer Society. *ACS Cancer Facts and Figures—2005*. Atlanta, GA: American Cancer Society; 2005.
2. Bernice M. Nursing care of the client with breast cancer. In: Itano JK, Taoka KN, eds. *Core Curriculum for Oncology Nursing*. 4th ed. St. Louis, MO: Elsevier Saunders; 2005:492-511.

3. Chapman DD, Moore S. Breast cancer. In: Yarbro CH, Frogge MH, Goodman M, eds. *Cancer Nursing: Principles and Practice*. 6th ed. Sudbury, MA: Jones and Bartlett; 2005:1022-1088.

4. Hogle WP, Quinn AE, Heron DE. Advances in brachytherapy: new approaches to target breast cancer. *Clin J Oncol Nurs*. 2003;7:324-328.

5. Kelly P, Levine M. *Breast Cancer: The Facts You Need to Know About Diagnosis, Treatment, and Beyond*. Buffalo, NY: Firefly Books; 2003.

6. Chu E, Devita V. *Cancer Chemotherapy Drug Manual*. Sudbury, MA: Jones and Bartlett; 2005: 102-106,141-145, 513-515, 181-186, 319-322.

7. In: Polovich M, White JM, Kelleher LO, eds. *2005 Chemotherapy and Biotherapy Guidelines and Recommendations for Practice*. 2nd ed. Pittsburgh, PA: Oncology Nursing Press; 2005:18-34.

8. Barse P, Calzone K, Dimond E, et al. Cancer risk assessment. In: Tranin A, Masny A, Jenkins J, eds. *Genetics in Oncology Practice*. Pittsburgh, PA: Oncology Nursing Society; 2001:75-130.

5

Chemotherapy-Induced Nausea and Vomiting Case Study

AB is a 19-year-old female diagnosed with osteogenic sarcoma coming to the clinic for her second cycle of chemotherapy. She is receiving cisplatin (Platinol) and doxorubicin (Adriamycin) every 21 days. AB is in good health. She has no past medical history, does not drink or smoke, and reports a history of motion sickness. When AB comes off the elevator to the clinic, she immediately runs into the bathroom. Her mother is accompanying her this morning and reports that she has been vomiting intermittently since she woke up this morning.

What might AB be experiencing?

She is experiencing anticipatory nausea and vomiting related to chemotherapy.

Why is it occurring?

Anticipatory nausea and vomiting occurs when a patient has experienced unrelieved nausea and vomiting with chemotherapy in the past. It is most likely due to stimulation of the limbic system, the part of the brain where memories live. Anticipatory nausea and vomiting is difficult to treat. This is why it is important to control nausea and vomiting from the beginning so that anticipatory nausea and vomiting does not develop.[1-2]

What interventions might help to prevent this type of nausea and vomiting in the future?

It is important to prevent or control any future chemotherapy-related nausea and vomiting. Benzodiazepines such as lorazepam (Ativan) 0.5 mg-1.0 mg IV or PO can be effective if taken the day of chemotherapy at home prior to arrival for chemotherapy. This can reduce anxiety, which is a risk factor of needing more aggressive antiemetic therapy.[1] Some patients also prevent anticipatory nausea and vomiting with behavioral modification strategies such as guided imagery, hypnosis, and biofeedback.

Would a pre-chemotherapy risk assessment have helped?

Yes, absolutely. If AB's nausea and vomiting had been prevented or controlled with the first cycle of chemotherapy, she might not have experienced anticipatory nausea and vomiting in subsequent cycles.[3] Acute emesis leads to anticipatory nausea and vomiting in 44% of patients. Chemotherapy-induced nausea and vomiting (CINV) can be devastating for patients with cancer.[4] Determination of the emetogenic risk of chemotherapy before treatment helps clinicians select the appropriate antiemetics and target teaching, as shown in **Table 5.1**.

What risk factors can be identified for AB related to chemotherapy-induced nausea and vomiting?

AB is a female less than 50 years old, she does not drink alcohol, and she has a history of motion sickness.[3] Her chemotherapy regimen is highly emetogenic.[2]

Table 5.1   **Emetogenic Risk by Antineoplast Agent**

High risk > 90%	Moderate risk 0%-90%	Low risk 10%-30%	Minimal risk < 10%
Carmustine > 250 mg/m^2	Carmustine < 250 mg/m^2	Aldesleukin (IL = 2)	Bleomycin
Cisplatin > 50 mg/m^2	Carboplatin < 250 mg/m^2	Asparaginase	Capecitabine
Cyclophosphamide > 1000 mg/m^2	Cyclophosphamide < 1000 mg/m^2	Docetaxel	Etoposide IV
Dacarbazine > 500 mg/m^2	Cyclophosphamide PO	Doxorubicin < 20 mg/m^2	Fludarabine
Dactinomycin	Cytarabine > 1 g/m^2	Etoposide PO	Methotrexate < 100 mg/m^2
Lomustine > 60 mg/m^2	Doxorubicin	Fluorouracil	Rituximab
Mechlorethamine	Epirubicin	Gemcitabine	Tenoposide IV
Pentostatin	Hexamethylmelamine	Methotrexate > 100 mg/m^2	Traztuzumab
Streptozocin	Idarubicin	Mitomycin C	Vinblastine
	Ifosfamide < 12 mg/m^2	Mitoxantrone Vinorelbine IV	
	Irinotecan	Paclitaxel	
	Melphalan	Temozolomide	
	Mitoxantrone > 12 mg/m^2	Thiotepa	
	Procarbazine	Topotecan	
	Oxaliplatin		

Source: Wilkes GM, Barton-Burke M, eds. Emetogenic risk by antineoplast agent. *2006 Oncology Drug Handbook.* Sudbury, MA: Jones and Bartlett; 2006:627.

What are some other risk factors that pertain to chemotherapy-induced nausea and vomiting?

Other risk factors include a history of nausea and vomiting with analgesic and/or anesthesia, history of hyperemesis with pregnancy, history of GI malignancy, radiation to the abdomen, history of anxiety or depression in the past, and prior inadequate control of nausea and vomiting.[3]

Nausea and vomiting have several different etiologies, as shown in **Figure 5.1**. The National Cancer Institute Common Toxicity Criteria helps clinicians determine the severity of nausea and vomiting (**Table 5.2**).

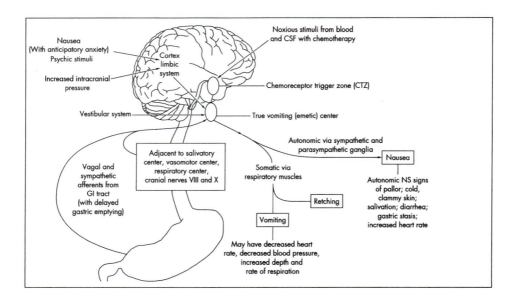

Figure 5.1   **The physiology of nausea and vomiting.**
Source: Reproduced from Barton-Burke MM, Wilkes GM, Ingwersen K, et al. *Chemotherapy and the Nursing Process.* Sudbury, MA: Jones and Bartlett Publishers; 1996:626. Drawing adapted from original by Gail Wilkes.

Table 5.2	**National Cancer Institute Common Toxicity Criteria: Nausea**				
	Grade				
Toxicity	*0*	*1*	*2*	*3*	*4*
Nausea	None	Able to eat	Oral intake significantly decreased	No significant intake, requiring IV fluids	—

Source: Wilkes GM, Barton-Burke M. *2005 Oncology Nursing Drug Handbook.* Sudbury, MA: Jones and Bartlett; 2005:1013.

What other types of nausea and vomiting exist that affect patients receiving chemotherapy?

In addition to anticipatory nausea and vomiting, there are acute, delayed, and breakthrough nausea and vomiting related to chemotherapy that we will discuss further as the case study progresses.

AB is given 0.1 mg intravenous lorazepam to help with the anticipatory nausea and vomiting after her port is accessed and blood is drawn for lab work. Other premeds include:

Palonosetron (Aloxi) 0.25 mg IV
Dexamethasone (Decadron) 12 mg IVP
Aprepitant (Emend) 125 mg PO 1 hour prior to chemotherapy on day 1 and 80 mg PO on days 2 and 3.

Briefly describe the classes of antiemetics listed previously and any side effects that AB could expect to experience.

Palonosetron is a serotonin antagonist but is different than the traditional agents in its class because it has a long half-life that makes it useful for delayed nausea and vomiting, which can occur after 24 hours and up to 6 days after chemotherapy administration. Palonosetron is effective in preventing acute nausea and vomiting in moderate and highly emetogenic chemotherapeutic regimens like cisplatin and is effective in preventing delayed nausea and vomiting in moderately emetogenic regimens.[1] Serotonin antagonists work by blocking the action of serotonin both centrally and peripherally. They are extremely effective in preventing acute nausea and vomiting. The original serotonin antagonists are ondansetron (Zofran), granisetron (Kytril), and dolasetron (Anzemet). Serotonin antagonists work best in combination with a corticosteroid such as dexamethasone for acute nausea and vomiting. Headache and constipation are the most commonly experienced side effects. Both of these side effects can be easily managed if a proactive approach is taken. Dexamethasone is a corticosteroid. In addition to working with serotonin antagonists, corticosteroids are used in combination with metoclopramide (Reglan) to treat delayed nausea and vomiting. Aprepitant is the first in a new class of antiemetics called the NK-1 receptor antagonists. It is an oral agent that crosses the blood-brain barrier. It works by blocking substance P, which is a tachykinin found in vagal afferent neurons that can cause nausea and vomiting by binding to the NK-1 receptors. It is very effective for acute and delayed nausea and vomiting associated with highly emetogenic agents. It must be given for 3 days and requires a serotonin antagonist and corticosteroid to be administered along with it. Aprepitant is very well tolerated. Side effects include hiccoughs and asthenia. Aprepitant (Emend) could significantly decrease international normalized ratio (INR) and affect the effectiveness of oral contraceptives. Doses of corticosteroids should be reduced by 50%.[1]

The rest of the visit proceeds uneventfully. AB receives prescriptions for lorazepam 1 mg po q 4 hours prn and prochlorperazine (Compazine) 10 mg po q 6 hours prn.

What other discharge instructions should AB receive related to CINV?

AB is asked to report any nausea and vomiting that is not relieved by her antiemetic regimen, especially if it lasts for more than 24 hours, because she is at risk for becoming dehydrated. This type of nausea and vomiting is called breakthrough emesis.[1]

In what class of antiemetics is prochlorperazine?

This antiemetic is a dopamine antagonist. The antiemetics in this class include metoclopramide and promethazine (Phenergan). Butyrophenones such as haloperidol (Haldol) also fall into this class. They bind to dopamine receptors in the brain, thereby blocking impulses to the vomiting center. They are helpful in preventing nausea and vomiting related to chemotherapy. These antiemetics cause sedation and extrapyramidal side effects. Extrapyramidal side effects can be relieved with diphenhydramine (Benadryl).[1]

What factors are important to consider when educating AB?

Readiness to learn and anxiety level should be assessed prior to beginning. Is she having any symptoms such as pain that would impair her ability to learn? Has she received any medications that would impair her ability to concentrate? Is the environment conducive to learning? Consider her reading level when providing written materials. Written materials should be geared to the layperson and in language that is readable to individuals with less than a high school education. The information should be reinforced, and a plan for this to occur should be in place.[5]

What type of instruction will AB receive?

AB's instruction should occur in a quiet, calm area. The plan for nausea and vomiting control should be clearly written out. AB should receive written materials about each antiemetic and about chemotherapy-induced nausea and vomiting to reinforce teaching.[5] AB must have a way to get her prescriptions from the pharmacy and be able to pay for them. If she has any anxiety about how she will be able to afford prescriptions, she might not be able to absorb any teaching. She might meet with the social worker or person who helps patients with financial issues first.

Three days later, AB's mother calls and says that her daughter has been experiencing ongoing nausea, has only been keeping sips of fluids down, and feels dizzy. Because AB is experiencing dizziness and is not keeping down fluids, further assessment is needed. She could be dehydrated. AB's mother should bring her daughter in for further assessment and possibly intravenous hydration and antiemetics.

What type of nausea and vomiting is AB experiencing and what interventions might be suggested?

This type of nausea is delayed nausea and vomiting and can commonly occur with regimens containing cisplatin, cyclophosphamide (Cytoxan), and carboplatin (Paraplatin).[1] It typically occurs 24 or more hours after chemotherapy and is experienced by 40%-50% of patients receiving emetogenic agents.[3]

AB's mother requests a copy of her daughter's electrolyte values. How should one respond to this request?

AB is 19 years old and is legally considered an adult. It is a privacy violation to share information without AB's prior consent. On the other hand, AB is an adolescent and it is important to encourage communication between mother and daughter. It would be appropriate to tell AB's mother that that information can be shared with her after obtaining permission from her daughter.

What nonchemotherapy cancer-related types of nausea and vomiting also exist?

Bowel obstruction, electrolyte imbalance, primary brain tumors or brain metastasis can also cause nausea and vomiting. These sources of nausea and vomiting should be considered in a patient undergoing chemotherapy who is experiencing unrelieved nausea and vomiting after receiving appropriate antiemetics.

REFERENCES

1. Vale PH. Integrating aprepitant and palonosetron into clinical practice: a role for new antiemetics. *Clin J Oncol Nurs.* 2005;9(1):77-84.

2. Hesketh PJ. Defining the emetogenicity of cancer chemotherapy regimens: relevance to clinical practice. *Oncologist.* 1999;4:191-196.

3. Doherty KM. Closing the gap in prophylactic antiemetic therapy: patient factors in calculating the emetogenic potential of chemotherapy. *Clin J Oncol Nurs.* 1999;3:113-119.

4. Grunberg SM, Devson RR, Mauros P, et al. Incidence of chemotherapy-induced nausea and emesis after modern antiemetics. *Cancer.* 2004;100:2261-2268.

5. Polovich M, White JM, Kelleher LO, eds. *2005 Chemotherapy and Biotherapy Guidelines and Recommendations for Practice.* 2nd ed. Pittsburgh, PA: Oncology Nursing Press; 2005:89.

6

Constipation Case Study

ES is a 35-year-old male diagnosed with non-Hodgkin's lymphoma coming in to the clinic for his first course of CHOP chemotherapy. Orders include:

Cyclophosphamide (Cytoxan) 750 mg/m^2 day 1

Doxorubicin (Adriamycin) 50 mg/m^2 day 1

Vincristine (Oncovin) 1.4 mg/m^2 (2 mg maximum dose) IVP day 1

Prednisone (Deltasone) 100 mg/day PO days 1-5

Premedications to prevent nausea and vomiting are included with his chemotherapy regimen; they include palonosetron (Aloxi) 0.25 mg IV and dexamethasone (Decadron) 12 mg IV, both 30 minutes prior to chemotherapy

ES had a left port placed 2 days ago. He reports that he is still taking 2 oxycodone and acetaminophen (Percocet) 5/325 tablets every 6 hours for pain. CS is in excellent physical condition, is very active, and plans to continue working as a hospital administrator.

Based on the data presented above, what 3 factors indicate that ES is at risk for developing constipation, and why?

Four of the medications—vincristine, palonosetron, oxycodone, and aceta-minophen—that ES is receiving can cause constipation. The physical mechanisms of constipation are related to decreased motility of the large intestine. Decreased motility can be caused by reduced strength of contraction within the intestines (peristalsis), poor muscle tone, and sensory changes within the anus and rectum. Vincristine causes autonomic nerve toxicity. It can also cause damage to the myenteric plexus of the colon. The patient may experience colicky abdominal pain or ileus.[1] Palonosetron is associated with constipation in about 5% of patients.[2] Opioids are the primary cause of medication-induced constipation.[1]

What are some other risk factors for developing constipation that cancer patients may have?

A cancer diagnosis such as ovarian or colon cancer in which a tumor or malignant ascites fluid could be pressing on and partially or totally occluding the bowel, intestinal or rectal surgery, radiation therapy to the abdomen, depression or anxiety, spinal cord compression involving the areas that innervate the bowel (anywhere from T8-L3), hypercalcemia, hypokalemia, dehydration, low fiber intake, overuse of laxatives, and preexisting metabolic, neurologic, or systemic conditions such as diabetes, stroke, Addison's disease, lupus, hypothyroidism, or hyperthyroidism. Even a change in environment or loss of privacy can predispose an individual to developing constipation.[1,3-4]

List some other medications that could cause constipation other than vinca alkaloid chemotherapy agents, opioids, and 5HT3 antagonist antiemetics.

Other medications causing constipation include non-steroidal anti-inflammatory drugs (NSAIDs), anticholinergics, diuretics, antacids containing aluminum or calcium, calcium or iron supplements, antihypertensives, tricyclic antidepressants, and anxiolytics.[1]

What should the nurse assess related to ES developing constipation?

ES's nurse should assess ES's patterns of elimination. When was his last bowel movement (BM)? ES should be asked about the color, volume, and consistency of stool and the presence of blood. A sudden onset of diarrhea could mean he has a severe impaction. Does he use laxatives and/or stool softeners? Has he experienced any changes in his living situation? His usual eating habits should be ascertained. Does he eat a diet high in fiber? Does he drink an adequate amount of fluids? Does he have any preexisting conditions? Does he already take any medications that can cause constipation? ES's functional status should be checked. Is he mobile? How active is he? The nurse should check his laboratory results for hypokalemia or hypercalcemia. His abdomen should be checked for symmetry, contour, distention, bulges, and peristaltic waves. Someone should listen to ES's bowel sounds in all 4 quadrants. Are they hyperactive or hypoactive? His abdomen should be palpated. Areas of increased resistance or tenderness should be sought. Finally, a physician, nurse practitioner (CRNP), or physician's assistant (PA) may perform a rectal exam as long as ES has an adequate white blood cell count and platelets. The physician, CRNP, or PA should check for fecal impactions, hemorrhoids, or fissures. Abdominal X-rays can be ordered if an ileus or obstruction is suspected, in order to differentiate between the two.[1,4]

What interventions are appropriate for ES to help prevent constipation from occurring?

Interventions are nonpharmacologic and pharmacologic. ES should be encouraged to increase fiber in his diet. Fiber helps increase transit time through the bowel. Fecal impaction occurs less frequently. Foods high in fiber include whole grain foods such as bran, fruits and vegetables, legumes, and nutritional supplements containing fiber. During the first few weeks that patients start increasing fiber in their diets, they may experience increased abdominal discomfort, flatulence, or erratic bowel habits. ES should be encouraged to gradually increase fiber over time and to drink at least 3 liters of fluid a day. Fluids can include items such as gelatin or soups. Warm fluids can stimulate a bowel movement. Caffeinated beverages and grapefruit juices act like diuretics and should be avoided. Preventative medical management usually involves a combination of a stimulating laxative combined with a stool softener, 1-2 tablets by mouth twice a day. ES should call office if he has not had a BM in 3 days.[1-2]

ES returns for a follow-up appointment and reports that he has not had a bowel movement in 3 days despite preventative interventions. What interventions should be suggested next?

The nurse instructs ES to take 3 bisacodyl (Dulcolax) tablets by mouth that evening. When she follows up the next day, she learns that ES did move his bowels.

Laxatives come in the following types: bulk-forming laxatives, saline laxatives, osmotic laxatives, detergent laxatives, and stimulant laxatives. Bulk-forming laxatives cause the stool to retain water and increase peristalsis. Laxatives in this category include fiber, bran, methylcellulose (Citrucel), and psyllium (Metamucil). Lubricants such as mineral oil coat and soften the stool so it can move more smoothly through the intestines. Saline laxatives pull water into the bowels and into the stool to increase peristalsis. Magnesium citrate, sodium biphosphate, and magnesium hydroxide are laxatives in this category. Osmotic laxatives work through bacteria in the colon that metabolize osmotic laxatives, causing an increased osmotic pressure gradient that pulls water into the intestines and then into the stool. The increased water increases peristalsis. Examples include glycerin suppository, lactulose (Cholac, Constilac, Constulose, Duphalac), and sorbitol. Detergent laxatives reduce the surface tension of the colonic cells so that water and fats enter the cell. Electrolyte and water absorption are decreased. The ducusate salts fall into this category. One example is ducusate calcium (Colace). Finally, stimulant laxatives irritate the intestines and increase motility. Senna (Senokot, Senexon) and bisacodyl fall into this category.[2]

Table 6.1   **National Cancer Institute Common Toxicity Criteria: Constipation**

			Grade		
Toxicity	*0*	*1*	*2*	*3*	*4*
Constipation	None	Requiring stool softener or dietary modification	Requiring laxative	Obstipation requiring manual evacuation or enema	Obstruction or toxic megacolon

Source: Wilkes GM, Barton-Burke M. *2005 Oncology Nursing Drug Handbook.* Sudbury, MA: Jones and Bartlett; 2005:1013.

If interventions did not relieve ES's constipation, what could happen?

ES could experience increased abdominal pain, decreased appetite, nausea and vomiting, and fecal impaction. More serious consequences could be ileus and bowel rupture with sepsis. Before any of these serious consequences occur, ES should be assessed for obstruction or impaction and his physician should be notified.[4] See also the National Cancer Institute Common Toxicity Criteria for constipation (**Table 6.1**).

REFERENCES

1. Polovich M, White JM, Kelleher LO, eds. *Chemotherapy and Biotherapy Guidelines.* 2nd ed. Pittsburgh, PA: Oncology Nursing Press; 2005:135-137.

2. Wilkes GM, Barton-Burke M. *Oncology Nursing Drug Handbook.* Sudbury, MA: Jones and Bartlett; 2005:608-609, 924-938.

3. Lynch MP. *Essentials of Oncology Care.* New York: Professional Publishing Group; 2005:132.

4. Kuck AW, Ricciardi L. Alterations in elimination. In: Itano JK, Taoka KN, eds. *Core Curriculum for Oncology Nursing.* 4th ed. St. Louis, MO: Elsevier Saunders; 2005:318-327.

Diarrhea Case Study

DJ is a 43-year-old male diagnosed with stage III colon cancer 2 months ago. He presented with blood in his stool and went to his primary doctor for a workup. A CAT scan revealed a mass in his sigmoid colon. He had a hemicolectomy 8 weeks ago and has recovered from this surgery without difficulty. DJ has a temporary colostomy. He comes to the clinic today for FOLFIRI with bevacizumab (Avastin). His chemotherapy regimen is as follows: irinotecan (Camptosar, CPT-11), fluorouracil (5-FU) bolus, leucovorin calcium (folinic acid) bolus, and fluorouracil (5-FU), continuous infusion over 46 hours and bevacizumab. He is receiving concurrent radiation therapy.

What factors indicate that DJ is at risk for developing diarrhea?

Up to 90% of patients undergoing chemotherapy and/or radiation therapy experience diarrhea. However, only 10%-30% of patients receiving chemotherapy alone experience chemotherapy-induced diarrhea. DJ's chemotherapy regimen, in particular, irinotecan and fluorouracil, puts him at high risk for developing diarrhea. Irinotecan is associated with early-onset and late-onset diarrhea. Early-onset diarrhea is associated with the cholinergic effects of the drug. DJ may experience diaphoresis and abdominal cramping preceding early-onset diarrhea. This can be effectively managed with atropine. About 88% of patients receiving irinotecan experience late-onset diarrhea. Late-onset diarrhea occurs 24 hours after the drug is taken and is relieved by loperamide (Imodium).[1] In addition, concurrent radiation to the abdomen and pelvis increases DJ's risk for developing diarrhea even more. Other chemotherapy agents associated with a high risk for developing diarrhea are: topotecan, paclitaxel (Taxol), dactinomycin (Actinomycin D, Cosmegen), and dacarbazine (DTIC). Some biotherapy agents also cause diarrhea. These include IL-2, interferons and monoclonal antibodies. Radiation to the abdomen, pelvis, or lower spine can lead to destruction of the cells of the lumen of the bowel.[2]

What could happen if chemotherapy- or biotherapy-related diarrhea is undertreated or left untreated?

There can be serious consequences. It can lead to dehydration, hospitalization, dose delays, dose reductions, and even death.[2] See also the National Cancer Institute Common Toxicity Criteria for diarrhea (**Table 7.1**).

What should DJ's nurse teach DJ and his family related to diarrhea?

DJ should learn to report signs and symptoms of acute diarrhea related to irinotecan such as sweating, abdominal cramping, and diarrhea during or after drug administration. He should receive atropine as ordered if acute-onset diarrhea occurs. For late-onset diarrhea, DJ should be instructed in self-management of diarrhea. This includes drinking 8-10 glasses of fluid a day, including broth, soda, and Gatorade, but avoiding milk products. He should also consume bland low-fiber foods and eat foods at room temperature. DJ should avoid foods that make diarrhea worse, such as fried, greasy, or spicy foods, raw fruits and vegetables, popcorn, beans, nuts, caffeine, and alcohol. The nurse should review DJ's medication list and instruct him to avoid taking any laxatives. DJ should begin loperamide 4 mg (two 2 mg capsules) at the first episode of diarrhea and then 2 mg (1 capsule) every 2 hours until diarrhea subsides. DJ should take 2 capsules (4 mg) at bedtime.

Table 7.1   **National Cancer Institute Common Toxicity Criteria: Diarrhea**

	Grade				
Toxicity	*0*	*1*	*2*	*3*	*4*
Diarrhea patients without colostomy:	None	Increase of < 4 stools/day over pretreatment	Increase of 4-6 stools/day, or nocturnal stools	Increase of < 7 stools/day or incontinence; or need for parenteral support for dehydration	Physiologic consequences requiring intensive care; or hemodynamic collapse
Patients with colostomy:	None	Mild increase in loose, watery colostomy output compared with pretreatment	Moderate increase in loose, watery colostomy output compared with pretreatment, but not interfering with normal activity	Severe increase in loose, watery colostomy output compared with pretreatment, interfering with normal activity	Physiologic consequences, requiring intensive care; or hemodynamic collapse

Source: Wilkes GM, Barton-Burke M. *2005 Oncology Nursing Drug Handbook.* Sudbury, MA: Jones and Bartlett; 2005:1013.

He should call if the diarrhea is not relieved by the loperamide or is bloody. His ability to purchase the antidiarrhea medication should be assessed prior to his going home. He should have loperamide on hand prior to starting chemotherapy with agents that cause diarrhea. If there is an anticipated problem, someone should assist him in finding alternate sources of obtaining the medications prior to sending him home.[2]

The most common types of chemotherapy diarrhea are osmotic, secretory, and exudative. Osmotic diarrhea occurs for 3 reasons: injury to the bowels, dietary factors such as lactose intolerance, and problems with digestion. All of these contribute to substances that the body cannot absorb that draw water into the intestines by osmosis, which, in turn, results in increased stool volume. This type of diarrhea is improved by eliminating the causative factor, such as glucose or lactose.[2] Secretory diarrhea occurs because there is an imbalance between absorption and secretion of fluids and electrolytes in the small and large intestines. Damage to the bowels can be caused by chemotherapy, radiation, or graft-versus-host disease. Other causes include infection and inflammation of the bowels and endocrine tumors. The imbalance between the absorption and secretion of fluids leads to a large volume of fluids and electrolytes in the small bowel. The colon cannot absorb it all and the end result is large volumes of diarrhea. This type of diarrhea is not relieved by fasting.[2] Exudative diarrhea occurs because of mucosal inflammation and ulceration caused by cancer treatment, cancer itself, and inflammatory diseases. When there are alterations in mucosal integrity and destruction of enzymes essential to carbohydrate and protein digestion, moderate to severe diarrhea could occur. If these changes are due to chemotherapy, the patient may experience diarrhea immediately and it could last for up to 14 days after.[2]

How should the nurse assess DJ related to diarrhea?

The nurse doing the assessment will first review DJ's history related to diarrhea. She would look at previous and current treatments for cancer, including all prescription and nonprescription medications. DJ's usual bowel pattern should be assessed, including frequency, color, amount, odor, and consistency of stool both currently and historically. Any recent changes in factors contributing to usual bowel elimination patterns should be noted, as should any change in life stressors or change from usual daily routine. She should check to see if DJ has started on any recent courses of antibiotics and look for recent dietary changes that increase bowel motility. This includes addition of fiber, fruit juices, caffeine, fried foods, and alcohol. Fluid intake should be reviewed. She should assess for the presence of flatus, abdominal bloating, cramping, pain, urgency, recent weight loss, and decreased urine output. She should note any weight loss greater than 1%-2% in a week. Also, she should note any indications of anxiety, fear, or complaints of social isolation.[3]

What should be noted as significant physical exam findings?

DJ should be assessed for the presence of hypotension, tachycardia, hyperactive bowel sounds, hard stool in the rectum, perineal skin irritation, poor skin turgor, and dry mucous membranes.[3]

What tests is the physician likely to order for DJ?

One can expect orders for stool culture for C. *difficile* x3 and serum electrolytes.[3]

DJ calls to report diarrhea the day after receiving his treatment, which is apparently late-onset diarrhea related to irinotecan. What can be done to intervene?

DJ can begin taking loperamide as described in the patient teaching section previously.

What could be done if the loperamide did not relieve the diarrhea that DJ was experiencing?

DJ could begin taking atropine and diphenoxylate hydrochloride (Lomotil) 5 mg po qid and then titrate to response for 2 days. The nurse should also instruct DJ to notify the physician if it is not effective.

What nonpharmacologic interventions can DJ learn related to diarrhea?

DJ should learn to maintain perineal cleanliness by thoroughly cleansing the area with mild soap, rinsing thoroughly, patting the area dry and applying a skin barrier after each bowel movement. He should weigh himself daily and report changes. Strategies such as relaxation, distraction, or imagery might help to modify stress response.[3]

Why is chemotherapy started at least 28 days after surgery before DJ receives bevacizumab?

Chemotherapy is started at least 28 days after surgery because bevacizumab is an angiogenesis inhibiter and DJ is at risk for bleeding. The surgical incision should be fully healed before the drug is started. If surgery is planned either after or during chemotherapy, bevacizumab should be stopped several weeks before surgery.[4]

REFERENCES

1. Wilkes GM, Barton-Burke M. *Oncology Drug Handbook*. Sudbury, MA: Jones and Bartlett; 2005:191-196.

2. Polovich M, White JM, Kelleher LO, eds. *Chemotherapy and Biotherapy Guidelines*. 2nd ed. Pittsburgh, PA: Oncology Nursing Press; 2005:118-123.

3. Kuck AW, Ricciardi L. Alterations in elimination. In: Itano JK, Taoka KN, eds. *Core Curriculum for Oncology Nursing*. 4th ed. St. Louis, MO: Elsevier Saunders; 2005:327-331.

4. Polovich M, White JM, Kelleher LO, eds. *Chemotherapy and Biotherapy Guidelines*. 2nd ed. Pittsburgh, PA: Oncology Nursing Press; 2005:50t.

8

End of Life Case Study

CF is a 46-year-old male who was diagnosed with advanced pancreatic cancer 9 months ago. He received 8 cycles of gemcitabine (Gemzar), which he tolerated very well. About 3 months ago, CF experienced a sense of constant fullness and nausea. A CT scan revealed disease progression, and CF elected to stop chemotherapy at that time. He has 3 children, ages 16, 14, and 10. CF was employed as a manager of a shoe store until the time of disease progression. He was introduced to the hospice team when he made the decision to stop chemotherapy and direct all efforts toward symptom management. A social worker opened his case and a plan was made for a primary nurse to see CF weekly. The number of visits were to be increased if CF's symptoms worsened. Three weeks ago, CF developed a bowel obstruction as evidenced by continuous vomiting, abdominal pain, bloating, and no BM for 6 days. A nasogastric (NG) suction tube was placed to decompress the bowel and make CF more comfortable. CF is currently receiving nothing by mouth except for sips of fluids and ice chips as needed for comfort. He was started 3 weeks ago on a fentanyl (Duragesic) patch 50 micrograms every 72 hours. CF currently reports his pain intensity as a 3 on a 0-10 pain scale, which he states is an acceptable level for him. He describes his pain as continuous, dull, crampy abdominal pain.

What are some benefits of early hospice intervention?

Hospice care provides a team-oriented approach to physical, emotional, and spiritual care for patients and families facing a life-threatening illness. Early referral allows for fuller use of the services available. Some services include physicians, home health aide, nurses, social workers, clergy, trained volunteers, and speech, occupational, and physical therapists. The patient and family direct goals of care. Care can be as aggressive as curative care, but has a focus on comfort, dignity, and quality of life. Benefits for CF and his family include early and proactive symptom management and anticipatory grief work with a social worker, chaplain, and bereavement counselor.[1]

What is the difference between hospice and palliative care?

The goals of both hospice and palliative care include aggressive symptom management to provide good quality of life. In many cases, the patient receiving palliative care is not at the end of his or her life. In fact, he or she might still be receiving active cancer treatment.

The primary nurse makes a visit and notes that CF has no bowel sounds as expected during the physical assessment. His mucous membranes are dry, but CF states he is comfortable with the ice chips. Pain intensity is as stated previously. The physical assessment is otherwise unremarkable.

What data is missing from the assessment?

Psychosocial and spiritual assessment is missing. How are CF and his family coping at this time in their lives?

CF has an advance directive that states he does not want any measures that could prolong his life, such as CPR, a feeding tube, or cardiac medications. CF also has a durable power of attorney for health care that designates his wife as the healthcare decision maker if he is not able to do so.

When does the advance directive go into effect?

The advance directive goes into effect when the patient is not capable of making his own decisions.[2]

What is the difference between a DNR order (do not resuscitate) and an advance directive?

A do not resuscitate order is an order written by a physician that states in the event of cardiac or respiratory arrest the patient should not be resuscitated. An advance directive is a statement of the patient's wishes in an event he or she is incapacitated. Each person's wishes are different; some patients will want heroic measures.[2]

What is the Patient Self Determination Act?

The Patient Self Determination Act was passed by the United States Congress in 1990. This legislation requires that all healthcare institutions receiving Medicare or Medicaid funds to ask all patients they admit if they have an advance directive. If a patient does not have an advance directive, the institution is required to provide information about it.[2]

What ethical principle does an advance directive support?

An advance directive supports the ethical principle of autonomy. The patient has a right to self-determination.[3]

CF's sister arrives from out of state. She has not seen CF in 3 years. She comes during a visit from the hospice nurse. She becomes very anxious and states "The lack of food and water is killing my brother. If you put in an IV everything will be fine."

How could the hospice nurse respond?

CF's sister's response to her brother's condition is a very common one, especially since she has not been present to see his gradual decline. Our society associates feeding with caring and it is very hard for family members not to do that. The hospice nurse can explain that CF's body is not able to tolerate fluids at this time. Fluids would actually make him more uncomfortable since the fluid would overload his circulatory system and it would cause edema in his extremities and other dependent areas. Breathing could be more difficult if fluid collected in his lungs and secretions would be more difficult to manage.[4]

What kind of interventions are appropriate for CF's children?

Age-specific counseling is appropriate for CF's children. This could include art therapy, music therapy, play therapy, and age-specific support groups.

CF becomes progressively weaker. He is no longer able to sit up in a chair during the day. A hospital bed is set up in his living room. The hospice nurse inserts a Foley catheter. The visiting nurse is now visiting 3 times a week and a nursing assistant comes for 4 hours a day on 3 alternate days of the week. His wife shares that CF has become increasingly more withdrawn and she is concerned.

How could the hospice nurse respond?

It is a normal part of the dying process for a person to become more withdrawn. CF may lose interest in his surroundings. Having someone else present is still important. CF may gain comfort from hearing his family's activity around him.[5]

The nursing assistant says that the skin on CF's hands, arms, legs, and feet looks blue and blotchy. The underside of the body appears darker. There is a bluish gray color around the mouth and paleness in the face. CF's skin is mottled. What might be happening?

CF is becoming mottled. Slow blood circulation causes mottling.[5]

Table 8.1	**End of Life Resources**

American Academy of Hospice and Palliative Medicine (AAHPM)
www.aahpm.org

Center to Advance Palliative Care (CAPC)
www.capc.org

Education in Palliative and End-of-life Care (EPEC)
www.epec.net

The End of Life Nursing Education Consortium (ELNEC)
www.aacn.nche.edu/ELNEC

End of Life/Palliative Education Resource Center (EPERC)
www.eperc.mcw.edu

Hospice Association of America
www.hospice-america.org

Hospice Education Institute/HospiceLink
www.hospiceworld.org

Hospice Foundation of America
www.hospicefoundation.org

Hospice Net
www.hospicenet.org

National Hospice and Palliative Care Organization
www.nhpco.org

What are other signs and symptoms that death is imminent?

CF may begin sleeping more as death becomes near. He may experience rattling sounds in the lungs and throat. This is known by some people as the "death rattle." This happens when the body loses its ability to clear secretions. The rattling does not indicate that the patient is uncomfortable. Suctioning at this time would cause discomfort and is not recommended. Caregivers can turn CF on his side and keep his mouth clean and moist. CF may become incontinent of urine and a Foley catheter is already in place. As less oxygen gets to the brain CF may become disoriented and restless. Caregivers should provide a calm environment and continue to be present. As the body continues to shut down, regular patterns of breathing change. Breathing can be rapid and shallow or there can be spaces between breaths.[5]

CF dies peacefully in his sleep. The hospice nurse comes to the house to pronounce his death.

What other types of follow-up care is appropriate for CF's family?

One of the benefits of hospice is follow-up bereavement support at regular intervals for the family.[1] A list of end of life resources can be found in **Table 8.1**.

References

1. Crowley MJ. Supportive care: dying and death. In: Itano JK, Taoka KN, eds. *Core Curriculum for Oncology Nursing*. 4th ed. St. Louis, MO: Elsevier Saunders; 2005:102-104.

2. Taylor-Johnson E. Spiritual and ethical end of life concerns. In: Yarbro CH, Frogge MG, Goodman M, Groenwald SL, eds. *Cancer Nursing Principles and Practice*. 5th ed. Sudbury, MA: Jones and Bartlett; 2000:1574-1575.

3. O'Connor KF. Ethical/moral experiences of oncology nurses. *Oncol Nurs Forum*. 1996;23(5):787-794.

4. Zerwekh JV. Do dying patients really need IV fluids? *Am J Nurs*. 1997;97(3):26-30.

5. North Central Florida Hospice, Inc. Preparing for approaching death. Available at: http://www.hospicenet.org/html/preparing_for.html. Accessed July 28, 2006.

9

AIDS-Related Lymphoma Case Study

SG is a 43-year-old male who presented to his primary medical doctor with several enlarged cervical lymph nodes, fever, night sweats, constipation, abdominal discomfort, and a 20-pound weight loss in the last 3 months. He was diagnosed with HIV 8 years ago and has been following up with his primary care doctor. A cervical lymph node biopsy confirmed the presence of high-grade diffuse large B-cell lymphoma. A non-Hodgkin's staging workup is scheduled.

What will SG undergo as part of the non-Hodgkin's lymphoma staging workup?

The staging workup for B-cell lymphoma consists of a complete history and physical, chest X-ray, blood counts and other blood studies, and abdominal-pelvic CT scans.[1] Patients who are diagnosed with HIV-associated lymphoma should also have a lumbar puncture to rule out central nervous system (CNS) involvement and baseline values for CD4 counts and viral load.[2]

The abdominal CT scan showed a large abdominal mass, the bone marrow biopsies were positive, and the blood counts were normal. SG is scheduled to receive CHOP (cyclophosphamide [Cytoxan], doxorubicin [Adriamycin], vincristine [Oncovin], and prednisone) chemotherapy the following week.

A nurse meets with SG in a pre-chemotherapy teaching session. She first assesses his coping skills. What does she assess?

She assesses his feelings about diagnosis and upcoming treatment, the coping strategies he has used in the past, and how well those strategies worked.[2]

She next assesses SG's social situation. What should she ask him?

She sensitively assesses his social support systems to determine if he has any transportation, economic, or insurance issues. SG may already have an established support system in place because of his HIV diagnosis. She should ask SG who his significant others are. His family of choice may be different than his family of origin. Determine who should receive what kind of information. The nurse should assess the need for durable power of attorney for health care and advance directive information and involve a social worker as needed.[3]

SG is enrolled in a Phase III clinical trial. What are the facility's responsibilities regarding clinical trials?

The facility must ensure that informed consent has been obtained and documented, that confidentiality is maintained, treatment responses and interventions are documented, symptoms are managed, patient selection is appropriate with phase criteria, and that the facility advocates as needed.[4]

SG asks how he can obtain more information about clinical trials. What should he be told?

Coalition of Cancer Cooperative Groups Trial Check is a search tool developed by the Coalition of Cancer Cooperative Groups to assist patients in locating clinical trials close to them. Information can be found at www.CancerTrialsHelp.org.

Describe the 4 phases of clinical trials and differentiate between the phases.

Each phase of clinical trials answers a different research question. They are conducted in a series of phases. Phase I clinical trials are conducted to test a new drug or treatment for the first time to identify safe dose ranges and side effects. Phase I trials usually involve a small group of participants. Phase II clinical trials involve a larger group of people. They are conducted to determine drug or treatment efficacy and safety. Phase III clinical trials involve an even larger number of participants. They are conducted to confirm the drug or treatment's effectiveness, compare it to commonly used treatments, and collect safety information. Phase IV studies are done after the drug or treatment is marketed to gather information about long-term side effects and additional information on the drug or treatment's effect on various populations.[5]

What function do the B lymphocytes have?

B cells are important to humoral immunity. They protect against bacteria and viral infections. When a B cell is stimulated, it produces plasma cells, which, in turn, produce antigen-specific antibodies.[3]

What is significant about B-cell lymphoma in the HIV population?

B-cell lymphoma is the most frequently diagnosed cancer in the HIV population.[3]

How does malignant disease occur as a result of HIV infection?

Immune surveillance function is already impaired and B cells are chronically stimulated. These two factors can result in cells that undergo malignant transformation.[3]

What are 3 factors that could make treating an HIV-infected individual more challenging?

Three factors that make treatment more challenging are that abnormal sites of cancer presentation are common, duration of response to treatment is poor, and patients may have opportunistic infections present at diagnosis or that develop during treatment.[3]

What are some risk factors for developing HIV-related lymphoma?

Risk factors include lower CD4 counts, usually below 200/mm[3], older age, and lack of highly active antiretroviral therapy (HAART).[3]

Should SG continue to take his HIV medications while receiving chemotherapy?[3]

Yes. HAART therapy should be given together with chemotherapy; however zidovudine (AZT) might cause bone marrow compromise.

SG receives his first dose of chemotherapy. What preventative measures related to infection are ordered?

Pegfilgrastim (Neulasta) and prophylactic antibiotics are ordered to help prevent neutropenic sepsis.

What symptoms should SG report related to neutropenic sepsis and opportunistic infection?

SG's nurse should teach SG to report temperature greater than 100.5°F, shortness of breath, cough, chest pain, mucositis, stomatitis, diarrhea, frequency or burning on urination, mental status changes, or skin rash.[3]

What factors are associated with a shorter survival when a person is diagnosed with HIV-related lymphoma?[3]

Such factors include CD4 counts below 100 cells/mm^3, stage III or IV disease, age older than 35 years, and elevated LDH.

What does LDH stand for and why is it significant?

LDH stands for lactate dehydrogenase and is a commonly known tumor marker. It is elevated in many cancers including lymphoma, seminoma, acute leukemia, and metastatic cancer. LDH is not used as a diagnostic tool because it is not a specific test for only one type of cancer. However, it can be very useful in monitoring treatment response. LDH is also elevated in nonmalignant conditions such as hepatitis and myocardial infarction.[6]

What is a normal LDH range?

A normal range is 100-215 U/I.[6]

What oncologic emergency is SG at risk for developing with his first chemotherapy cycle based on the amount of disease present at diagnosis?

SG is at risk for developing tumor lysis syndrome (TLS).[7]

What is TLS?

TLS is a metabolic oncologic emergency that occurs because tumor cells are being killed rapidly. It develops because potassium, phosphorus, and nucleic acid are being rapidly released into the bloodstream. It is characterized by hyperkalemia, hyperphosphatemia, and hyperuricemia, which happens when nucleic acid converts to uric acid, and by hypocalcemia, which occurs because the increased amount of phosphorus binds to calcium and forms calcium phosphate salts.[7] See also **Table 9.1**.

Table 9.1   **Tumor Lysis Syndrome**

Early signs and symptoms	Late signs and symptoms	Nursing measures
Hypocalcemia	Acute renal failure	Maintain aggressive hydration
Hyperkalemia	Seizures	Strict I/O
Hyperphosphatemia	Cardiac arrest	Daily weights
Hyperuricemia		Monitor daily labs
		Check for signs and symptoms of overload

Source: Gobel BH. Metabolic emergencies. In: Itano JK, Taoka KN, eds. *Core Curriculum for Oncology Nursing.* 4th ed. St. Louis, MO: Elsevier Saunders; 2005:395-400.

If SG develops TLS, is it serious?

Yes, it is potentially life threatening. Cardiac arrhythmia, kidney failure, or multiple organ failure can occur.[7]

What interventions can be begun during and after the first chemotherapy treatment to help prevent TLS?

SG can begin aggressive hydration with normal saline or dextrose prior to beginning prechemotherapy and continuing posttreatment. The hydration can be infused at 150-200 ml/hr. Urine output will also be 150-200 ml/hr. Urine alkaline should be kept to decrease the solubility of uric acid and prevent renal damage. The urine PH should be tested with each void and kept above 7. Oral or intravenous sodium bicarbonate may be added as needed. Allopurinol (Zyloprim) can be administered as ordered, either oral or intravenous to decrease uric acid production. Strict intake and output should be maintained and SG should be weighed daily. Calcium, potassium, phosphorus, and uric acid should be monitored carefully.[7]

What should be done if urine output is not 150-200 ml/hr?

The physician should be notified; if hydration is adequate, a loop diuretic might be ordered, and if that is not effective, mannitol might be ordered.[7]

What is one potential complication that could occur if a loop diuretic is used?

Dehydration might occur.[7]

What are some additional preventative strategies?

SG should avoid oral potassium or phosphorus supplements, dietary sources of possasium and phosphorus, and nephrotoxic medications.[7]

REFERENCES

1. Iwamoto RR. Nursing care of the client with lymphoma or multiple myeloma. In: Itano JK, Taoka KN, eds. *Core Curriculum for Oncology Nursing.* 4th ed. St. Louis, MO: Elsevier Saunders; 2005:689-700.

2. Zelenentz AD, Advani RH, Buadi F, et al. The NCCN non-Hodgkins lymphoma clinical practice guidelines oncology. *J Natl Comprehensive Cancer Network.* 2006;14(3):258-310.

3. Moran TA. Nursing care of the client with HIV-related cancers. In: Itano JK, Taoka KN, eds. *Core Curriculum for Oncology Nursing.* 4th ed. St. Louis, MO: Elsevier Saunders; 2005:716-735.

4. Nelson-Martin P, Glover JJ. Selected ethical issues in cancer care. In: Itano J, Taoka K, eds. *Core Curriculum for Oncology Nursing.* 4th ed. St. Louis, MO: Elsevier Saunders; 2005:909-920.

5. National Library of Medicine, U.S. National Institutes of Health. Glossary of clinical trials terms. Available at: http://www.clinicaltrials.gov/ct/info/glossary. Accessed July 30, 2006.

6. Camp-Sorrell D, Hawkins RA. Tumor markers. In: Camp-Sorrell D, Hawkins RA, eds. *Clinical Manual for the Oncology Advance Practice Nurse*. Pittsburgh, PA: Oncology Nursing Press; 2000;1011-1022.

7. Gobel BH. Metabolic emergencies. In: Itano JK, Taoka KN, eds. *Core Curriculum for Oncology Nursing*. 4th ed. St. Louis, MO: Elsevier Saunders; 2005: 395-400.

10

Hypercalcemia Case Study

WZ is a 73-year-old African American female diagnosed 6 years ago with multiple myeloma. She was treated with VAD chemotherapy and her disease remained relatively stable until 1 month ago. She had not been receiving any treatment and has maintained a good quality of life. Today she presents to the outpatient clinic complaining of lethargy, weakness, back pain, nausea, and decreased appetite. She states that her pain is 6 on the 0-10 pain scale. WZ states that it has begun to interfere with her ability to perform her normal daily activities. She is the caregiver of 3 grandchildren while her daughter works during the day. WZ has a past medical history of hypertension and diabetes.

What is multiple myeloma?

Multiple myeloma is a cancer of the bone marrow. It is a malignancy of the plasma cells that produce immunoglobins. These particular cancer cells make abnormal proteins that can build up in the body. Normal plasma cells are an important part of the immune system. The cancer cells collect in the bone marrow and in the hard outer part of the bones. Sometimes they collect in only one bone and form a single tumor. Usually they collect in many bones, forming many tumors. This is the reason it is called multiple myeloma. Multiple myeloma usually occurs between the ages of 50 and 70. It is more prevalent in the African American population. Median time from diagnosis to death is 10 years. Most patients die of the disease or the complications.[1]

What does VAD stand for and why did WZ receive this type of therapy?

VAD stands for vincristine (Oncovin), doxorubicin (Adriamycin), and dexamethasone (Decadron).[2] It is the most common chemotherapy treatment used for multiple myeloma. This regimen has less risk of myelosuppression (anemia, neutropenia, and thrombocytopenia) than protocols containing alkylating agents. This is a good treatment choice for WZ because of her age and comorbidities.

What oncologic emergency is WZ experiencing based on her presenting symptoms?

WZ presented with lethargy, back pain, weakness, nausea, and decreased appetite. These are all signs and symptoms of hypercalcemia.[3]

What is the normal function of calcium in the body?

Calcium is necessary for proper maintenance of healthy bones, teeth, tissue, muscle, and nerve functioning. It helps maintain normal clotting mechanisms, converting prothrombin to thrombin.[4]

What is a normal calcium range?

A normal range is 8.5-11 mg/dl. Mild hypercalcemia is a calcium level greater than 11 mg/dl, moderate hypercalcemia is 12-14 mg/dl, severe hypercalcemia is 14-16 mg/dl, and any level greater than 16 mg/dl is considered life threatening hypercalcemia.[5]

What is hypercalcemia?

Hypercalcemia is the most common oncologic emergency. It occurs in 10%-20% of all patients with cancer.[3] It can be life threatening in some patients. A serum calcium level above 11 mg/dl is considered hypercalcemic. Hypercalcemia is a metabolic disorder that results in a syndrome of increased bone resorption caused either by bone destruction, related tumor invasion, increased secretion of parathyroid hormone, osteoclast activating factor, or prostaglandin produced by

Table 10.1	Incidence of Hypercalcemia in Particular Malignancies	
Malignancy	**Reported Incidence**	**References**
Lung		3,11,16
Squamous cell	35%	
Other	11%	
Breast	17%-40%	8,16
Hematologic		10,15,16
Multiple myeloma	20%-40%	
Lymphoma	<10%	
Genitourinary	12%	16
Head and neck (squamous)	2.5%-25% (varies by site)	9,16
Renal cell	6%	7
Unknown primary	7%	7
Liver (primary)	3%	7,16
Other: cholangiocarcinoma, clear cell carcinoma of the ovary, pancreatic islet cell, vipoma	1%	8,12
Prostate, uterine, colorectal, primary bone, parathyroid, chronic lymphocytic leukemia, chronic myelogenous leukemia, acute leukemia, small cell lung cancer	<1%	8,13-16

Source: Yarbro CH, Frogge MH, Goodman M, Groenwald S, eds. *Cancer Nursing Principles and Practice.* 6th ed. Sudbury, MA: Jones and Bartlett; 2005:792.

cancer cells. Normal levels of calcium in the body are regulated by parathyroid hormone. It stimulates release of calcium from bone when bloodstream calcium levels fall. The gastrointestinal tract is responsible for absorption of vitamin D. Proper kidney function is needed for excretion of calcium. The kidneys normally handle the excretion of calcium but cannot keep up with the amount of calcium in hypercalcemia.[5]

Ninety percent of patients who develop hypercalcemia have breast cancer, lung cancer, head and neck cancer, multiple myeloma, renal cancer, lymphoma, or primary hyperparathyroidism. The incidence varies widely depending on tumor type.[5]

For what early signs and symptoms of hypercalcemia should WZ be assessed?

Early signs and symptoms of hypercalcemia include fatigue, weakness, brady-cardia, arrhythmias, apathy, confusion, personality changes, confusion, anorexia, constipation, nausea and vomiting, weight loss, bone pain, and renal calculi.[5]

What are some late signs and symptoms of hypercalcemia for which WZ should be assessed? Does WZ exhibit any of these signs and symptoms?

Currently WZ does not have any late signs and symptoms of hypercalcemia. They include heart block, cardiac arrest, stupor, coma, ileus, and renal failure.[5]

What diagnostic tests are ordered for WZ? Describe additional tests that can be used in the assessment of hypercalcemia.

Tests for serum calcium, potassium, magnesium, sodium, and albumin are routinely ordered when hypercalcemia is suspected, and these are the tests that are ordered for WZ. Albumin is checked because decreased albumin could create a false normal calcium level. In addition to elevated calcium, one should look for decreased serum sodium, magnesium, and potassium. BUN and creatinine tests are ordered when dehydration is present. Serum phosphorus and alkaline phosphatase tests are ordered if bony involvement is suspected. Immunoreactive

Table 10.2   **Manifestations of Hypercalcemia Associated with Cancer**

Organ System	Signs and Symptoms
Neurological	
Central nervous system	Altered cognition Confusion Apathy Drowsiness or lethargy Pain **Late:** Obtundation, coma
Peripheral neuromuscular	Muscle weakness Hypotonia Decreased respiratory muscle capacity Decreased or absent deep-tendon reflexes
Renal	Polyuria Dehydration (dry mucous membranes, orthostatic hypotension, etc.) Occasional nephrocalcinosis
Cardiovascular	Prolonged P-R interval Widened QRS Shortened QT, ST intervals Bradycardia (with rapid increases) **Late:** Widened T-waves, broadened T-wave, heartblock, ventricular arrhythmias, asystole Enhanced sensitivity to digitalis Hypertension (if intravascular volume is maintained)
Gastrointestinal	Increased gastric acid secretion Anorexia Nausea and vomiting Constipation Acute pancreatitis (rare) **Late:** Obstipation

Source: Yarbro CH, Frogge MH, Goodman M, Groenwald S, eds. *Cancer Nursing Principles and Practice.* 6th ed. Sudbury, MA: Jones and Bartlett; 2005:799.

parathyroid hormone levels are ordered to distinguish hyperparathyroid hypercalcemia from malignant hypercalcemia. Levels will be decreased or undetectable in cancer-related hypercalcemia. An EKG could be ordered depending on the potassium level.[5] A CT scan of the spine is ordered for WZ because of her back pain.

WZ has normal blood test results with the exception of her calcium level that was 14 mg/dl. The CT scan revealed an L4 lesion.

What treatment options are available to treat WZ's hypercalcemia?

Several options are available for the treatment of hypercalcemia. These include hydration, diuretics, bisphosphonates, and chemotherapy or radiation to treat the underlying cancer.[5]

WZ is admitted to the hospital and the following orders are written:

Normal saline solution (NSS) at 125 ml/hour
Zoledronic acid (Zometa) 4 mg IV over at least 15 minutes
Dexamethasone 60 mg IV every 6 hours
Oxycodone with acetaminophen (Percocet) 5/325 mg 2 tablets every 4 hours
    prn pain
Prochlorperazine (Compazine) 10 mg IV every 6 hours prn nausea
Senna (Senokot, Senexon) 2 tablets bid
Encourage oral fluid intake
Radiation consultation
Physical therapy consultation

What is the rationale for each order?

The normal saline IV is ordered to correct dehydration and increase renal excretion of calcium. WZ has moderate hypercalcemia based on her calcium level of 14 mg/dl. Aggressive hydration is important to prevent or minimize renal damage. It should continue for at least 48 hours unless WZ's cardiac status indicates otherwise. The rationale is the same for increasing oral fluid intake. The effect of hydration alone is only temporary. Zoledronic acid is a third-generation bisphosphonate used to

Table 10.3   **Focused History for Suspected Hypercalcemia**

Focus	Comments
Chief complaint/reason for seeking care	Most commonly neurological/mental status symptoms, but maybe other symptom(s) of advanced cancer, GI symptom, pain, polyuria, etc.
Symptom(s)	
Onset/duration	Recent onset or long-standing symptoms?
Progression	Rapid or slow worsening of symptoms?
Severity	Patient's rating.
Associated symptoms	If patient does not volunteer, ask about frequent urination, thirst, constipation (ask if patient is taking an opioidanalgesic), weakness, fatigue.
Effects on important ADLs, QOL	Altered ambulation, nightmares.
Diagnosis of cancer confirmed?	Is this a malignancy in which hypercalcemia occurs?
Known bone metastases?	Breast cancer and multiple myeloma are frequently associated with hypercalcemia.
Previous episodes of hypercalcemia	Associated with increased risk for occurrence.
Current therapy for cancer	
Chemotherapy	Can therapy be the cause of some of the symptoms?
New estrogen or antiestrogen	Has bone pain increased with new hormone (may indicate tumor flare)?
Medications	Ask about over-the-counter medications and alternative/ complementary supplements in addition to prescription drugs.
Megavitamins	
Nutritional supplements	Do CV assessment; report bradycardia or irregular HR to MD;
Calcium	hold digoxin until after consulting with MD.
Vitamin A, D	
Shark cartilage	
Thiazide diuretic	
Lithium	
Digoxin	
Other	Ask about:
	Activity level, especially bed rest

(*continues*)

Table 10.3	Focused History for Suspected Hypercalcemia (*continued*)
Focus	**Comments**
	Whether pain, nausea/vomiting, or other unrelieved symptoms interfere with activity
	Current/usual appetite and diet
	Weight loss in last 6 months; calculate percent weight loss (>10% may indicate protein/calorie malnutrition).

GI = gastrointestinal; ADL = activities of daily living; QOL = quality of life;
CV = cardiovascular; HR = heart rate; MD = physician.

Source: Yarbro CH, Frogge MH, Goodman M, Groenwald S, eds. *Cancer Nursing Principles and Practice.* 6th ed. Sudbury, MA: Jones and Bartlett; 2005:801.

treat cancer-induced hypercalcemia. Bisphosphonates work by binding to mineralized bone matrix and preventing calcium phosphate crystal dissolution. They are both effective and easy to tolerate. Dexamethasone is a corticosteroid used to treat steroid-sensitive cancers such as multiple myeloma and lymphoma. WZ reports a moderate level of pain that can be relieved with a narcotic analgesic. Prochlorperazine is ordered to treat WZ's nausea. Treating symptoms such as pain and nausea can help to increase mobility. Oxycodone and acetaminophen is ordered for WZ's back pain. Senna is ordered to prevent constipation related to oxycodone with acetaminophen. Radiation therapy to the lesion in WZ's lumbar spine will help relieve the back pain as well. Physical therapy is ordered because exercise and weight-bearing activities are important components of maintaining bone mass.[5]

What happens if zoledronic acid is administered more quickly than over 15 minutes?

This drug will cause renal dysfunction with the rise in serum creatinine if it is given too quickly. This can be dangerous in a patient who already has the potential for kidney dysfunction due to hypercalcemia. Calcium clears through the kidneys.[2]

What else can be done if WZ does not respond to these treatments or if her hypercalcemia progresses to severe or life threatening?

Peritoneal dialysis or hemodialysis can be started. These are also used for patients who have congestive heart failure or renal insufficiency and cannot tolerate saline hydration.[5]

List 5 nursing diagnoses that pertain to WZ.

Nursing diagnoses that pertain to WZ include risk for injury, deficient fluid volume, risk for constipation, nausea, and altered nutrition that is less than body requirements.[5]

What should WZ's nurse teach WZ in preparation for radiation therapy?

Her nurse should teach WZ that radiation is a local treatment. Side effects of radiation depend on the area being radiated and the length of time radiation will last. She is going to be radiated to the lumbar spine region. She could expect to experience skin changes in the radiation field and fatigue. She could possibly experience nausea, vomiting, and diarrhea.[6]

What other nursing measures can be implemented for WZ?

The nurse should maximize safety while WZ is in the hospital. He should make sure her call light is within reach and her bed is locked and in the low position. He should implement seizure precautions when the calcium level is above 12 mg/dl. He must maintain strict intake and output, including maintenance of urine output between 100 and 150 ml/hour. He should weigh WZ daily and encourage mobility and do range of motion exercises while she is in bed. WZ's nurse should monitor her for changes in neurovascular status and manage symptoms of nausea, pain, and constipation. WZ should not take multivitamins or antacids containing calcium.[5]

WZ stays in the hospital for 5 days and feels progressively better each day. Her serum calcium is now 9 mg/dl. She is reporting decreased pain—now 3 on the 0-10 pain scale. WZ is now ambulating without difficulty.

What discharge instructions should WZ receive?

WZ and her family should be informed about signs and symptoms of hypercalcemia to report. She must have a good understanding of the follow-up schedule, including appointments for blood work and seeing the medical oncologist. WZ has some remaining radiation treatments, so it is important to determine if there will be any barriers such as transportation issues to completing treatment. WZ should try to remain physically active. WZ should report an increase in pain, particularly since it will be a barrier to adequate mobility.[4-5]

REFERENCES

1. American Cancer Society. Multiple myeloma. 2006. Available at: http://www. cancer.org/docroot/CRI/content/CRI_2_4_1X_What_is_multiple_myeloma_ 30.asp. Accessed August 2, 2006.

2. Wilkes GM, Barton-Burke M. *2005 Oncology Nursing Drug Handbook*. Sudbury, MA: Jones and Bartlett Publishers; 2005:707-710, 1097.

3. National Cancer Institute. Hypercalcemia (PDQ®) Health Professional Version. 2006. Available at: http://www.cancer.gov/cancertopics/pdq/supportive-care/hypercalcemia/HealthProfessional. Accessed on June 8, 2006.

4. Smith WJ. Hypocalcemia/hypercalcemia. In: Camp-Sorrell D, Hawkins RA, eds. *Clinical Manual for the Oncology Advance Practice Nurse*. Pittsburgh, PA: Oncology Nursing Press; 2000:849-858.

5. Gobel BH. Metabolic emergencies. In: Itano JK, Taoka KN, eds. *Core Curriculum for Oncology Nursing*. 4th ed. Philadelphia, PA: Saunders Elsevier Company; 2005:400-406.

6. American Cancer Society. *Understanding Radiation Therapy: A Guide for Patients and Families*. Author; 2004:27.

7. Harvey HA. The management of hypercalcemia of malignancy. *Support Care Cancer* 3:123-129, 1995.

8. Raue F. Epidemiological aspects of hypercalcemia of malignancy. In: Raue W, ed. *Recent Results in Cancer Research*. Berlin: Springer-Verlag; 1994:99-106.

9. Muggia FM. Overview of cancer-related hypercalcemia: epidemiology and etiology. *Semin Oncol* 1990;17(Suppl 5):3-9.

10. Mosekilde L, Eriksen EF, Charles P. Hypercalcemia of malignancy: pathophysiology, diagnosis and treatment. *Crit Rev Oncol Hematol* 1991;11:1-27.

11. Warrell RP. Etiology and current management of cancer-related hypercalcemia. *Oncology* 1992;6:37-43.

12. Orloff JJ, Stewart AF. Disorders of serum minerals caused by cancer. In: Coe FL, Favus MJ, eds. *Disorders of Bone and Mineral Metabolism*. New York: Raven; 1992:539-561.

13. Mao C, Carter P, Schaefer P, et al. Malignant islet cell tumor associated with hypercalcemia. *Surgery* 1995;117:37-40.

14. Brown EM, Harris HW, Vassilev PM, et al. The biology of the extracellular Ca^{2+}-sensing receptor. In: Bilezikian JP, Raisz LG, Rodan GA, eds. *Principles of Bone Biology*. New York: Academic; 1996, 243-262.

15. Roodman GD. Mechanisms of bone metastasis. *Cancer* 80:1557-1563, 1997.

16. Heys SD, Smith IC, Eremin O. Hypercalcemia in patients with cancer: aetiology and treatment. *Eur J Surg Oncol* 1998;24:139-143.

11

Mucositis Case Study

TM is a 72-year-old male who was in his usual state of health until he noticed a worsening hoarseness 5 months ago. Three weeks ago he began to have trouble swallowing, which got progressively worse. He now is only able to swallow soft foods. TM reports a 10-pound weight loss in the past 3 months. He reports no change in appetite. He states that his level of fatigue is increasing and he now requires frequent rest periods. TM has undergone extensive evaluation of these symptoms, including a CT scan and biopsy. The CT scan revealed a left supra-glottic tumor. Left-sided adenopathy was also noted. Biopsy confirmed squamous cell carcinoma. TM is married and has 2 grown children. He tells his nurse his wife is very supportive and will accompany him to his appointments. He says he is a retired printer and that he owned his own printing business. TM currently smokes 50 cigarettes a day. He reports heavy alcohol use in the past. A head and neck surgeon, a radiation oncologist, and a medical oncologist evaluated him. TM has been advised that he will need both chemotherapy and radiation treatments. The chemotherapy regimen is cisplatin (Platinol) on days 1, 22, and 43 of radiation treatments. He is at the outpatient oncology clinic for his first cycle of chemotherapy. Radiation is scheduled daily for a total of 6 weeks. A PEG feeding tube was placed 2 days ago to be used if it is needed. The dietitian will see TM while he is at the clinic for chemotherapy.

What side effect is TM at great risk for developing because he will be receiving radiation to the head and neck and concurrent chemotherapy?

TM is at great risk for developing oral mucositis.

What characterizes oral mucositis?

Oral mucositis is characterized by inflammation and ulceration of the mucous membranes.[1]

How common is oral mucositis?

Approximately 40% of patients receiving standard dose chemotherapy, 80% of patients undergoing hematopoietic stem cell transplantation, and 100% of patients receiving radiation therapy for cancer of the head and neck with or without chemotherapy experience oral mucositis. This is why TM will receive proactive care from the beginning of treatment and why he must be monitored carefully for the presence of oral mucositis.[1]

What is oral mucosal tissue composed of?

Oral mucosal tissue contains stratified squamous nonkeritinized epithelium, followed by the submucosa, which contains the blood and nerve supply, inflammatory cells, and the extracellular matrix.[1]

Why is it important to understand normal mucosal physiology?

A nurse who understands normal physiology and the expected changes that occur with mucositis will be better equipped to detect changes.[1]

In addition to concurrent radiation and chemotherapy what risk factors does TM have for developing oral mucositis?

Known risk factors so far are TM's age and smoking history. Risk factors for developing oral mucositis can be divided up into 2 categories, individual risks and treatment-related risks. Individual risk factors include age, gender, nutritional status, oral hygiene, salivary function, and genetics.[1]

Individuals who are older than 50 experience oral mucositis that is more severe and lasts longer than those who are younger than 50 do. This is potentially due to normal decline in renal function, which affects how chemotherapy is excreted. Women experience oral mucositis more often than men. Individuals with poor nutrition are more prone to oral mucositis. Poor nutrition leads to deficiencies in vitamins and trace elements, which affect the regenerative power of the mucous membranes.[2]

Patients who have poor oral hygiene, poor-fitting dentures, or those who smoke, drink alcohol, or eat spicy foods are at increased risk due to irritation of the mucous membranes, which may already be present. Preexisting reduced salivary flow or xerostoma will also increase the risk of oral mucosa.[2]

Chemotherapeutic agents that are associated with increased risk of developing oral mucositis include (in addition to cisplatin); vinorelbine (Navelbine), gemcitabine (Gemzar), doxorubicin (Adriamycin), docetaxel (Taxotere), paclitaxel (Taxol), fluorouracil (5-FU), methotrexate, and cyclophosphamide (Cytoxan).[3]

What will prechemotherapy oral assessment include?

The nurse should check TM for ill-fitting dentures, potentially irritating teeth surfaces, preexisting gingivitis, or infection. She should check the mucosal tissue for any changes in color, such as pallor or erythema. Note that TM has preexisting hoarseness and unintentional weight loss.[2]

Should TM have dental work done while receiving chemotherapy or radiation?

No, all dental work should be done prior to chemotherapy.[1]

What are the 5 steps in the process of developing mucositis?

Mucositis does not just appear; there are actually 5 steps in the process. The first step is the initiation phase. This occurs when radiation or chemotherapy damage DNA. This damage results in mucosal cell, tissue, and blood vessel damage. The next phase is the upregulation and generation of messenger signals. Proinflammatory cytokines that are responsible for tissue injury and programmed cell death are released. Then the signaling and amplification phase occurs. The proinflammatory cytokines activate the production of more cytokines that alter the structure of mucosal tissues. Once this has happened, the ulceration phase occurs. Ulcers penetrate through the epithelium to the submucosa. Bacteria penetrate the submucosa and stimulate macrophage activity. This further increases the release of proinflammatory cytokines. Angiogenesis is stimulated. Finally, the healing phase occurs. Epithelial proliferation occurs until the mucosa returns to normal thickness. Tissues do not return to complete normalcy, however. This is why someone who has had 1 episode of mucositis is at increased risk for injury in the future.[1]

Is there a standard of care for the prevention and treatment of oral mucositis?

No. Currently no standard of care exists. However, the goals of treatment include providing symptom relief and preventing further mucosal damage.[2] Clinical practice guidelines were issued in 2004 by the Multinational Association for Supportive Care in Cancer (MASCC) along with the International Society for Oral Oncology (ISOO). The guidelines suggested that oral care protocols, including patient education, should be instituted in an attempt to reduce the severity of oral mucositis. Their recommendations are the most reliable to date.[4] The importance of preparing a patient at risk for developing mucositis about what to expect cannot be underestimated. Patients who are well prepared can better manage and tolerate side effects.[5]

What preventative measures could be instituted for TM?

TM can begin an oral hygiene program after meals and at bedtime. TM should brush with a soft toothbrush and change to a sponge swab if he becomes neutropenic or thrombocytopenic. He should rinse his mouth with saline or baking soda, using a vigorous swish. TM should avoid oral irrigators because they could force microorganisms into compromised areas, leading to infection. He should avoid irritating agents such as commercial mouthwashes, hot or spicy foods, alcohol, tobacco, and lemon glycerin swabs.[2]

Should TM suck on ice chips prior to his chemotherapy to also help prevent oral mucositis?

Having a patient suck on ice chips appears to work for bolus chemotherapy such as bolus fluorouracil (5-FU), but is not recommended for infusional chemotherapy.[4]

What other measures are used to help prevent oral mucositis?

They are divided into 2 categories; medications used to lessen or improve the severity of oral mucositis and topical or systemic medications used to manage pain. Medications used to improve or lessen oral mucositis include allopurinol (Zyloprim), amifostine (Ethyol), benzydamine, and chlorhexidine (Peridex). One small study done in 1994 showed that allopurinol mouthwash had a statistically significant improvement in the prevention of oral mucositis. The sample size was small and the study needs to be replicated. Amifostine is an antioxidant in the radiation treatment field that has protective qualities on oral mucosa. It can be given either as a subcutaneous injection or as an intravenous infusion. The optimal dose for protection against mucositis has not been determined. Side effects include headaches, nausea, rash, and orthostatic hypotension. Side effects appear to be more severe when the drug is given intravenously. Benzydamine is recommended in the MASCC/ISOO guidelines for the prevention and treatment of oral mucositis in cancer patients. One barrier is that it is not yet available to patients in the United States. It is currently available in Canada and Europe. It is applied as a topical mouthwash. It has analgesic, antimicrobial, anesthetic, and anti-inflammatory effects. Chlorhexidine is a broad-spectrum antibiotic mouth rinse that is used to manage plaque-dependent oral mucositis. MASCC/ISOO guidelines do not recommend its use based on clinical trials that show that chlorhexadine does not prevent the development of oral mucositis in patients with head and neck cancer undergoing radiation.[4]

What are the possible clinical consequences of oral mucositis for TM?

TM could experience chemotherapy dose reductions, treatment delays, infection, changes in nutrition, extra clinic visits for pain management or hydration, increased morbidity and mortality and a negative impact on his quality of life.[3]

Three weeks into treatment TM calls and complains of increased difficulty swallowing, pain, and ulcers in his mouth. He is now only able to swallow liquids. He also complains "nothing tastes the same." What should the nurse tell him?

TM is asked to come into the clinic to have these symptoms evaluated because it is difficult to evaluate mucositis over the phone. Most likely he will need some further interventions.

What phase of mucositis is TM experiencing?

TM is experiencing the ulcerative phase.[1]

TM comes into the clinic for evaluation. How should the nurse assess his oral mucosa?

First the nurse should examine the lips, tongue, and oral mucosa for color, moisture, integrity, and cleanliness. If TM was wearing dentures or other dental appliances, she should be sure to ask him to remove them. Then she should assess TM for changes in taste, voice, ability to swallow, and the presence or absence of pain during swallowing. TM should rate the severity of pain on a 0-10 linear scale if he is able. This will provide consistency when the nurse assesses the symptom, and in the future it will allow her to know if any of her interventions have helped. Then she should examine the saliva for amount and quality. Is it thick, ropy, copious in amount, etc.? Is TM's mouth dry? She should ask TM when the symptoms started and check for anything that aggravates or relieves the symptoms.[2] **Table 11.1** is a useful grading criteria that can help nurses accurately describe the severity of mucositis.

What else does the nurse assess?

TM may be dehydrated or be experiencing a decline in nutritional status, so his nurse needs to check skin turgor, orthostatic vital signs, and current weight against baseline. The nurse should also ask TM about oral intake.[2]

Based on the assessment, the nurse determines that TM is experiencing moderate mucositis.

What changes could be made to the oral hygiene program that was started prior to treatment?

If oral mucositis is mild to moderate, oral hygiene should be increased to every 2 hours. If it is severe, the program should be increased to every hour.[2]

Is the pain that occurs with oral mucositis somatic, visceral or neuropathic?

Acute pain that is associated with oral mucositis is somatic in nature. Mechanisms include stimulation of the nociceptors in the mucosal tissue and the inflammatory process.[6]

Table 11.1   National Cancer Institute Common Toxicity Criteria: Mucositis

Gastrointestinal Toxicity						
		Grade				
Adverse event	Short name	1	2	3	4	5
Mucositis/stomatis (clinical exam) - Select - Anus - Esophagus - Large bowel - Larynx - Oral cavity - Pharynx - Rectum - Small bowel - Stomach - Trachea	Mucositis (clinical exam) - Select	Eyrthema of the mucosa	Patchy ulcerations or pseudo-membranes	Confluent ulcerations or pseudo-membranes; bleeding with minor trauma	Tissue necrosis; significant spontaneous bleeding; life-threatening consequences	Death
Remark: Mucositis/stomatitis (functional/symptomatic) may be used for mucositis of the upper aerodigestive tract caused by radiation, agents of GVHD.						
Mucositis/stomatis (functional/symptomatic) -Select - Anus - Esophagus - Large bowel - Larynx - Oral cavity - Pharynx - Rectum - Small bowel - Stomach - Trachea	Mucositis (functional/symptomatic) Select	*Upper aerodigestive tract sites:* Minimal symptoms, normal diet; minimal respiratory symptoms but not interfering with function *Lower GI sites:* Minimal discomfort, intervention not indicated	*Upper aerodigestive tract sites:* Symptomatic but can eat and swallow modified diet; respiratory symptoms interfering with function but not interfering with ADL *Lower GI sites:* Symptomatic, medical intervention indicated but not interfering with ADL	*Upper aerodigestive tract sites:* Symptomatic and unable to adequately aliment or hydrate orally; respiratory symptoms interfering with ADL*Lower GI sites:* Stool incontinence or other symptoms interfering with ADL	Symptoms associated with life-threatening consequences	Death
Nausea	Nausea	Loss of appetite without alteration in eating habits	Oral intake decreased without significant weight loss, dehydration or malnutrition; IV fluids indicated < 24 hrs	Inadequate oral caloric or fluid intake; IV fluids, tube feedings, or TPN indicated 24 hrs	Life-threatening consequences	Death
Also consider: Anorexia, vomiting.						

Source: From National Cancer Institute Common Toxicity Criteria, Version 3.0 [Online] revised December 12, 2003. Available at: http://ctep.cancer.gov/reporting/ctc_v30.html. Accessed November 6, 2006.

What treatment might TM receive?

If TM is exhibiting signs and symptoms of dehydration, he may receive 1 to 2 liters of fluids in the office if it cannot be replaced utilizing the feeding tube. One immediate goal will be to lessen the severity of the pain TM is experiencing. A pain management regimen will be started. Agents used to manage pain related to oral mucositis fall into 2 categories: topical anesthetics and systemic analgesics.[6]

What topical agents are available, and when are they used?

Topical agents are mainly used for mild to moderate oral mucositis pain (0-6 on the 0-10 linear pain scale). Topical anesthetics provide local pain control without systemic side effects. Pain relief from topical agents is short in duration—usually 1-2 hours or less. Agents that are used topically include lidocaine (Xylocaine viscous), sucralfate (Carafate), Magic Mouthwash, morphine mouthwash, and Gelclair. Xylocaine viscous acts as a local anesthetic and is taken 10-15 minutes before eating. Some patients have difficulty with the viscousness of the solution itself or the whole-mouth-numbing effects. One way around the whole-mouth-numbing effects is to have the patient use a cotton-tipped swab and apply the solution to affected areas only. This works well if mucositis or mouth ulcers are not throughout the entire oral mucosa. Sucralfate suspension works by forming a protective coating on mucosal tissue. It may stimulate the production of prostaglandin E2 that has protective effects on mucosal tissue and increases blood flow and production of mucus. Magic Mouthwash has many different components that vary from institution to institution. Some combinations can include diphenhydramine hydrochloride (Benadryl), calcium carbonate (Maalox), and tetracycline (Mycostatin). This approach can contain medications that have side effects of their own and is not evidence based. Morphine mouthwash may work because of upregulation of peripheral opioid receptors in tissue inflammation. Gelclair is a bioadherent oral gel that is FDA approved as a medical device instead of a drug and requires a prescription for its use. It has moisturizing and lubricating properties. It works by forming an adherent barrier over the oral mucosa that protects exposed or sensitized nerves. Patients mix 1 packet of Gelclair with 15 ml of water and rinse their mouths with it and spit it out after a minute. Patients should not eat or drink for 1 hour after use.[6]

How are systemic analgesics used in the treatment of oral mucositis?

Opioids are generally used for moderate to severe oral mucositis pain (6-10 on the 0-10 linear pain scale) because of their systemic effects. Systemic pain relief lasts longer than topical pain relief. The World Health Organization recommends morphine as the opioid of choice for managing severe pain. The regimen is tailored to the patient. Managing the pain may involve a combination of long- and short-acting agents. If oral medications do not work, other routes must be considered. For example, the MASCC/ISOO guidelines recommend PCA morphine as the treatment of choice in the hematopoietic stem cell transplant setting. Nonopioid analgesics such as NSAIDs can help along with opioids to systemically treat pain and reduce tissue damage from inflammation.[6]

How will TM's nutritional needs be addressed?

If TM does not have sufficient oral intake, tube feedings need to be initiated. Ideally, TM will have been shown how to use and maintain the tube prior to actually needing it. This strategy will make the transition much smoother.

TM continues tube feedings and is able to complete both chemotherapy and radiation. He reports no further weight loss and has even gained a pound. How long after treatment is completed will tube feedings be necessary?

Because the mucosal epithelium takes 7-14 days to regenerate, tube feedings will continue for at least 2 weeks after treatment has been completed and all tissues have healed. Some patients will require much longer than this, especially patients who have received radiation.[1]

What are some additional nursing measures that are important in TM's treatment of mucositis?

Being present and providing emotional support is an important nursing function. It has a positive effect on patients and families. Support must continue after therapy has been completed because oral mucositis may still be present after therapy is completed.[5]

REFERENCES

1. Van Gerpen RA. Overview of mucositis. *Oncol Supportive Care Q.* 2005;3(2):4-9.

2. Polovich M, White JM, Kelleher LO, eds. *2005 Chemotherapy and Biotherapy Guidelines and Recommendations for Practice.* 2nd ed. Pittsburgh, PA: Oncology Nursing Press; 2005:89.

3. Peterson DE. New strategies for the management of oral mucositis in cancer patients. *J Supportive Oncol.* 2006;4(2):9-13.

4. Brown CG. Where do we go from here? The evidence-based approach to the treatment of oral mucositis. *Oncol Supportive Care Q.* 2005;3(2):11-17.

5. Armstrong JA, McCaffrey R. The effects of mucositis on quality of life in patients with head and neck cancer. *Clin J Oncol Nurs.* 2006;10(1):53-56.

6. Bruce SD. Pain management issues and strategies in oral mucositis. *Oncol Supportive Care Q.* 2005;3(2):18-27.

12

Neutropenic Sepsis Case Study

CS is a 73-year-old female recently diagnosed with non-Hodgkin's lymphoma. She was treated with CHOP/rituximab (Rituxan) 1 week ago. This is her first cycle of chemotherapy.

What should a nurse teach CS in preparation for discharge following this first cycle of chemotherapy?

A nurse should instruct CS to report a temperature greater than 100.5°F, shaking chills, shortness of breath, unusual bruising or bleeding, burning or frequency when urinating, nausea, vomiting, or diarrhea that lasts more than 24 hours, constipation lasting greater than 48 hours, and redness, tenderness, or induration around her venous access device insertion site.[1] The nurse also gives CS written information for her and her family to review at home to reinforce teaching.

What are the risk factors related to the development of neutropenic sepsis?

Risk factors include age 65 or older, treatment with a chemotherapeutic regimen with a greater than or equal to 40% risk of febrile neutropenia, extensive previous treatment with chemotherapy, or radiation to the sites where bone marrow is produced, tumor invasion of the bone marrow, hematologic malignancy, poor performance status, multiple comorbidities, history of febrile neutropenia, decreased immune function, open wounds, elevated LDH (non-Hodgkin's lymphoma), and serum albumin greater than 3.5 (non-Hodgkin's lymphoma).[2-3] **Figure 12.1** is an example of a pre-treatment risk assessment tool.

Does CS have an increased risk of developing neutropenic sepsis? Please explain.

Yes, non-Hodgkin's lymphoma is a hematologic malignancy, CS's chemotherapeutic regimen is myelosuppressive, and her age is greater than 65.

What preventative measures can be taken?

A nurse will teach CS to avoid all invasive tests and procedures unless absolutely necessary beginning a week to 10 days postchemotherapy, since any break in the body's first line of defense, the skin and mucous membranes, could cause infection. Her nurse instructs her to maintain excellent oral hygiene using a soft toothbrush and rinsing with saline (1 teaspoon of salt to a quart of water) or baking soda (1 teaspoon of baking soda to 1 cup of water) 5 times a day. CS should be given a prescription for a stool softener and she should be advised that straining with a stool could result in trauma to the rectal mucosa. She should be instructed to use a stimulating laxative such as senna concentrate (Senokot) if she does not have a bowel movement within 2 days.[1] Her nurse teaches her about safe food-handling precautions. This means that CS should avoid uncooked meat or fish, thaw meat in the refrigerator, carefully handle eggs, avoid stagnant water, wash fruits and vegetables carefully, and avoid buffets or salad bars. The neutropenic diet may be implemented if a patient becomes febrile and is hospitalized or is undergoing stem cell or bone marrow transplantation. In most cases, the diet consists of the components of safe food handling, and in addition, no fresh fruits and vegetables unless they are first washed and peeled. The neutropenic diet is currently a controversial subject; the body of evidence still needs to be developed and guidelines vary from institution to institution.[4-5] CS should be encouraged to

AIMhigher
Assessment. Information. Management.

Pre-Treatment Risk Assessment

Page 1 of 2

Patient: _____ Diagnosis: _____

Regimen: _____ Date: _____

NEUTROPENIA

- ○ Myelosuppressive Chemo Regimen
- ○ Hx of Severe and/or Febrile Neutropenia
- ○ Pre-existing Neutropenia
- ○ Extensive Prior Chemotherapy
- ○ Previous/Concurrent Radiation to Marrow

- ○ Advanced or Uncontrolled Cancer
- ○ Bone Marrow Involvement
- ○ Poor Nutritional Status (e.g., low albumin)
- ○ Poor Performance Status (ECOG ≥ 2)

- ○ Elevated LDH (NHL)
- ○ Active Tissue Infection
- ○ ↓ Immune Function (consider other co-morbidities)
- ○ Other _____

- ○ Open Wounds
- ○ Age > 65

Risk identified? _____ Comments: _____

CHEMOTHERAPY REGIMENS ASSOCIATED WITH INCREASED TOXICITY

Bladder Cancer
paclitaxel/cisplatin or carboplatin
methotrexate/vinblastine/doxorubicin/cisplatin (MVAC)
Breast Cancer
docetaxel/doxorubicin (TA)
docetaxel/doxorubicin/cyclophosphamide (TAC)
doxorubicin/paclitaxel (AT)
AC→T, AC
Cervical
paclitaxel/cisplatin

Head & Neck
paclitaxel/ifosfamide/mesna/cisplatin
Non-Hodgkin's Lymphoma
cyclophosphamide/doxorubicin/vincristine/prednisone (CHOP)
dexamethasone/cisplatin/cytarabine/prednisone (DHAP)
etoposide/methyprednisolone/cisplatin/cytarabine (ESHAP)
Non-Small Cell Lung Cancer
cisplatin/paclitaxel
docetaxel/carboplatin
Testicular Cancer
vinblastine/ifosfamide/cisplatin (VIP)

Ovarian Cancer
paclitaxel
docetaxel
topotecan
Small Cell Lung Cancer
etoposide/cisplatin
topotecan+/-paclitaxel
Sarcoma
doxorubicin/ifosfamide
mesna/doxorubicin/ifosfamide/dacarbazine (MAID)

▪ This list is not comprehensive. Other regimens are associated with intermediate or high risk of febrile neutropenia.
▪ Consider CSF in regimens administered with curative/adjuvant intent (to maintain Relative Dose Intensity – RDI).

ANEMIA

- ○ Myelosuppressive Chemo Regimen
- ○ Bone Marrow Involvement
- ○ Nutritional Deficiency/Malabsorption

- ○ Previous Radiation to Marrow
- ○ Blood Loss–Surgical, GI, GYN
- ○ Transfusion Within Past 6 Months

- ○ Active Infection
- ○ Chronic Illness
- ○ Other _____

- ○ Renal Insufficiency
- ○ Pre-existing Anemia

Risk identified? _____ Comments: _____

CHEMOTHERAPY REGIMENS ASSOCIATED WITH INCREASED TOXICITY

cisplatin/5-FU
cyclophosphamide/doxorubicin/5 FU
cyclophosphamide/doxorubicin/vincristine/prednisone (CHOP)

cyclophosphamide/mitoxantrone/vincristine (CNOP)
etoposide/cisplatin
paclitaxel/cisplatin or carboplatin

paclitaxel/doxorubicin
topotecan

NAUSEA / VOMITING

- ○ Emetogenic Treatment Regimen
- ○ Female
- ○ < 50 years
- ○ Hx of N/V with Anesthesia/Analgesics

- ○ Radiation to Abdomen
- ○ Hx of Hyperemesis with Pregnancy
- ○ GI malign and/or Adv / large Tumor Burden

- ○ Prior Inadequate Control of N/V
- ○ Hx of Motion Sickness
- ○ Other _____

Risk identified? _____ Comments: _____

CHEMOTHERAPY REGIMENS ASSOCIATED WITH INCREASED TOXICITY

Intermediate Risk (occurs in at least 30% of patients)

amifostine > 500mg/m²   oxaliplatin > 75mg/m²
arsenic trioxide   procarbazine
etoposide   teniposide
gemcitabine   topotecan
interleukin-2 12-15 mil units/m²
irinotecan
melphalan > 500mg/m²
mitomycin
mitoxantrone

High Risk (occurs in >30% to 90% of patients)

busulfan > 4 mg/day   epirubicin
carboplatin   hexalmethylmelamine
carmustine   idarubicin
cyclophosphamide   ifosfamide
cytarabine   lomustine
dacarbazine   mechlorethamine
dactinomycin   methotrexate > 1000mg/m²
daunorubicin   streptozocin
doxorubicin

Very High Risk (occurs in 99% of patients)
cisplatin

The health care provider utilizing this form assumes all risks associated with its use.

Figure 12.1   Supportive Oncology Services Multi-symptom Risk Assessment tool

AiMhigher

Pre-Treatment Risk Assessment   Page 2 of 2

ANXIETY / DEPRESSION

○ Chemotherapy/Other Rx
○ Pancreatic, Brain, GYN, Lung, H&N Cancer
○ Relapsed/Refractory Disease
○ Uncontrolled Pain

○ Personal or Family Hx of Anxiety/Depression
○ Drug or Alcohol Abuse
○ Impaired Sexual Function
○ Altered Physical Appearance

○ Loss of Social/Emotional Support
○ Loss of Financial Resources
○ Loss of Functional Abilities
○ Other _____

Risk identified? _____   Comments: _____

CHEMOTHERAPY REGIMENS ASSOCIATED WITH INCREASED TOXICITY

asparaginase	interleukin	procarbazine	vinblastine
interferon	intrathecal methotrexate	tamoxifen	vincristine

ORAL MUCOSITIS

○ Chemotherapy
○ Current or Prior Radiation to H&N Area
○ Hx of Mucositis
○ Hx or Presence of Dental Disease

○ ↓ Salivation
○ Geriatric Patient
○ Poor Fitting Oral Prosthesis
○ Other _____

Risk identified? _____   Comments: _____

CHEMOTHERAPY REGIMENS ASSOCIATED WITH INCREASED TOXICITY

5-FU	dactinomycin	doxorubicin	methotrexate	thioguanine
bleomycin	daunorubicin	etoposide	mitoxantrone	vinblastine
cytarabine	docetaxel	floxuridine	plicamycin	

CONSTIPATION

○ Chemotherapy   ○ Geriatric Patient
○ Hx of Constipation ○ Current Narcotic Use
○ Antiemetics   ○ Oral Iron
○ Inactivity   ○ Other _____

Risk identified? _____

Comments: _____

CHEMOTHERAPY REGIMENS ASSOCIATED WITH INCREASED TOXICITY

thalidomide	vincristine
vinblastine	vinorelbine

DIARRHEA

○ Chemotherapy   ○ Enteral Feedings
○ Radiation to Colon/Abd/Pelvis ○ Lactose Intolerance
○ Hx of Diarrhea/Bowel Disease   ○ Other _____

Risk identified? _____

Comments: _____

CHEMOTHERAPY REGIMENS ASSOCIATED WITH INCREASED TOXICITY

5-FU	erlotinib	irinotecan
docetaxel	gefitinib	oxaliplatin

- **Neurotoxicity** – high-dose cyclophosphamide, high-dose cytarabine

- **Peripheral Neuropathy** – bortezomib, carboplatin, cisplatin, docetaxel, oxaliplatin, paclitaxel, paclitaxel protein-bound, thalidomide, vinblastine, vincristine, vinorelbine

- **Cardiac Toxicity** – doxorubicin, epirubicin, liposomal doxorubicin, mitoxantrone, traztuzumab

- **Hand and Foot Syndrome** – capecitabine, liposomal doxorubicin

Other Toxicities to Consider: _____

Signature: _____

The health care provider utilizing this form assumes all risks associated with its use.

Figure 12.1   **Supportive Oncology Services Multi-symptom Risk Assessment tool** (*continued*)

use a moisturizing skin lotion if dry skin occurs to help maintain skin integrity. In addition, CS should shave with an electric razor. One of the main ways that infection can be prevented in the healthcare setting is careful hand washing by all staff who come in contact with CS. Meticulous site care should be given to all central and peripheral catheter sites. If CS is hospitalized, invasive procedures such as rectal temperatures and suppositories, Foley catheters, nasogastric tubes or subcutaneous or intramuscular injections should be avoided (growth factor injections are acceptable). If hospitalized, CS, like other neutropenic patients, should wear a mask when leaving the floor her room is on for tests and procedures. The nurse should encourage mobility, and if that is not possible, she should encourage coughing, turning, and deep breathing and range of motion.[1] She could also give CS an incentive spirometer.

Should growth factors be used on the first cycle of CS's regimen?

According to the 2006 NCCN guidelines for myeloid growth factors in cancer treatment, growth factors such as filgrastim (Neupogen) and pegfilgrastim (Neulasta) should be ordered for regimens that have a greater than 20% risk (high) of developing febrile neutropenia, other neutropenic events, or compromising treatment. Growth factors should be considered for patients who have a moderate risk (10%-20% for these conditions). According to NCCN guidelines, CS's regimen falls into the 10%-20% range, so growth factors should be considered. Remember, CS has other risk factors that include age and a hematologic malignancy.[5]

What are the assessment criteria for neutropenic sepsis?

The nurse instructs CS to take her temperature at home if she feels warm. It is important to make sure she has a thermometer at home. A neutropenic patient in the hospital should have her vital signs, especially temperature, taken every 4 hours. It is important to know that if a neutropenic patient says she is chilly or has shaking chills, she could be becoming septic, in which case the fever will rise shortly after the shaking chill. The nurse should be extra alert for this situation. She should instruct CS to report oral mucositis, ulcers, or white patches, cough, sore throat, cloudy urine, burning or frequency when urinating, and hematuria. Skin and central or peripheral catheter sites should be inspected daily by CS or her caregiver. Redness, swelling, induration, and exudates like pus are often absent in patients with neutropenia, but fever, pain, and erythema will be present. If CS is hospitalized in addition to the above assessment criteria, her nurse should monitor white blood cell (WBC) and absolute neutrophil count (ANC) values daily, assess lungs every 4 hours, inspect skin of all body sites with high potential for infection such as mouth, skin folds, buttocks, perineum, axilla, central and peripheral catheter sites, and bone marrow biopsy sites every shift. Note changes in behavior such as restlessness, irritability, inappropriate euphoria, changes in level of consciousness and orientation, or headache. These neurological changes can all be early signs of impending sepsis.[1]

CS was instructed to go to the emergency room (ER) if her temperature exceeds 100.5°F. She arrives in the ER at 7 pm today and is being admitted to the oncology floor.

Vital signs: Temperature 103°F, pulse 128, respirations 32, and blood pressure 90/60.

Counts: hemoglobin 7.9, hematocrit 23, white blood cells 0.2 mm^3, platelets 36, segs 20%, bands 5%. She appears warm and flushed but reports having an uncontrollable shaking chill 2 hours ago.

What are the signs and symptoms of neutropenic sepsis?

CS has a fever, is tachycardic, tachypneic, and slightly hypotensive. All of these are early signs and symptoms of septic shock. Hypotension will occur more profoundly as cool shock approaches. Skin will be warm and flushed initially and peripheral cyanosis and cold, clammy extremities are seen as shock advances. Other signs and symptoms include decreased urine output progressing to anuria and changes in mental status. A physician must assess the patient as soon as possible, preferably in the early stages of sepsis. Nurses might need to be advocates for the patient in this situation.[1]

Calculate the absolute neutrophil count (ANC). Please note if CS is neutropenic.

$$\% \text{ segs} + \% \text{ bands} = \text{TNC (total neutrophil count)}$$
$$\text{TNC} \times \text{WBC (cells/mm}^3) = \text{ANC (cells/mm}^3)$$

Note: when calculating the ANC, percent is changed to a decimal and WBC is multiplied by 100 since the WBC is listed in mm³.

$$0.20 + .05 = .25$$
$$0.25 \times 200 = 50$$

According to Fishbach's definition of neutropenia,[6] CS is severely neutropenic. **Table 12.1** is a useful grading criteria that can help nurses accurately describe the severity of neutropenia.

Discuss what immediate nursing actions the nurse should take for CS.

The nurse would get an order to obtain aerobic and anaerobic blood cultures, either peripherally and through the central venous catheter, or from 2 separate peripheral sites; urine culture and sensitivity; throat, sputum, and skin cultures as appropriate; and a chest X-ray. According to the 2004 NCCN guidelines for fever and neutropenia, antibiotics need to be administered promptly at the first

---

Table 12.1   **National Cancer Institute Common Toxicity Criteria: Neutropenia**

Neutrophils/granulocytes/ANC

ANC ≥ 1500 ≤ 2000/mm³ – Grade 1
ANC ≥ 1000 ≤ 1500/mm³ – Grade 2
ANC ≥ 500 ≤ 1000/mm³ – Grade 3
ANC < 500/mm³ – Grade 4

Source: Wilkes GM, Barton-Burke, M. *2005 Oncology Nursing Drug Handbook.* Sudbury, MA: Jones and Bartlett; 2005:988.

sign of infection (i.e., fever).[7] IV fluids will be hung. Normal saline may be initially instituted.

What other nursing measures are used to manage neutropenic sepsis?

Continued frequent assessment, monitoring vital signs, and monitoring of intake and output.[1]

Differentiate between the hyperdynamic (warm shock) and the hypodynamic (cool shock) phases of septic shock.

Early Signs and Symptoms of Septic Shock
Normal or elevated temperature
Chills
Warm, flushed skin
Anorexia
Normal or low blood pressure

Hyperdynamic Phase (Warm Shock)
Normal or elevated temperature
Chills and rigors
Restlessness
Changes in level of consciousness (anxiety, confusion, restlessness)
Tachycardia
Bounding pulses
Widening pulse pressure
Decreased urine output

Hypodynamic Phase (Cool Shock)
Subnormal temperature
Disorientation and lethargy
Hypotension
Tachycardia

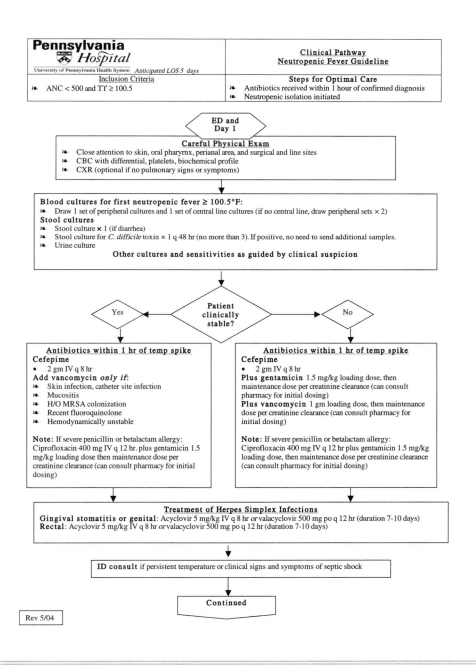

Figure 12.2   Pennsylvania Hospital neutropenic fever pathway.

Source: Provided courtesy of Pennsylvania Hospital.

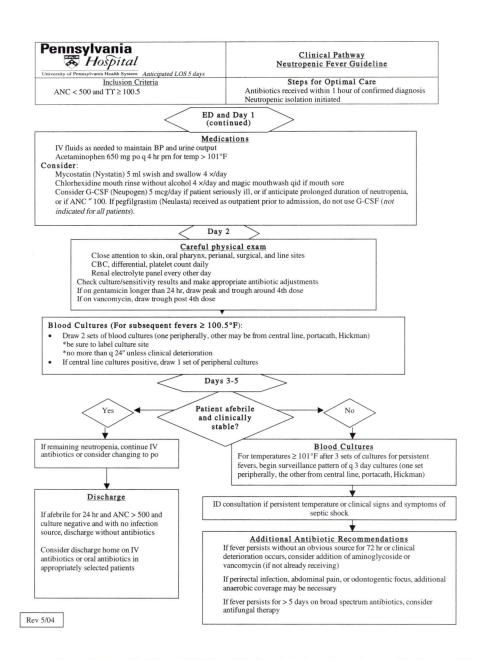

Pennsylvania *Hospital*
University of Pennsylvania Health System *Anticipated LOS 5 days*

**Clinical Pathway
Neutropenic Fever Guideline**

Inclusion Criteria	Steps for Optimal Care
ANC < 500 and TT ≥ 100.5	Antibiotics received within 1 hour of confirmed diagnosis
Neutropenic isolation initiated

**ED and Day 1
(continued)**

Medications
IV fluids as needed to maintain BP and urine output
Acetaminophen 650 mg po q 4 hr prn for temp > 101°F
Consider:
Mycostatin (Nystatin) 5 ml swish and swallow 4 ×/day
Chlorhexidine mouth rinse without alcohol 4 ×/day and magic mouthwash qid if mouth sore
Consider G-CSF (Neupogen) 5 mcg/day if patient seriously ill, or if anticipate prolonged duration of neutropenia, or if ANC ″ 100. If pegfilgrastim (Neulasta) received as outpatient prior to admission, do not use G-CSF (*not indicated for all patients*).

Day 2

Careful physical exam
Close attention to skin, oral pharynx, perianal, surgical, and line sites
CBC, differential, platelet count daily
Renal electrolyte panel every other day
Check culture/sensitivity results and make appropriate antibiotic adjustments
If on gentamicin longer than 24 hr, draw peak and trough around 4th dose
If on vancomycin, draw trough post 4th dose

Blood Cultures (For subsequent fevers ≥ 100.5°F):
- Draw 2 sets of blood cultures (one peripherally, other may be from central line, portacath, Hickman)
  *be sure to label culture site
  *no more than q 24° unless clinical deterioration
- If central line cultures positive, draw 1 set of peripheral cultures

Days 3-5

Patient afebrile and clinically stable?

Yes

If remaining neutropenia, continue IV antibiotics or consider changing to po

Discharge
If afebrile for 24 hr and ANC > 500 and culture negative and with no infection source, discharge without antibiotics

Consider discharge home on IV antibiotics or oral antibiotics in appropriately selected patients

No

Blood Cultures
For temperatures ≥ 101°F after 3 sets of cultures for persistent fevers, begin surveillance pattern of q 3 day cultures (one set peripherally, the other from central line, portacath, Hickman)

ID consultation if persistent temperature or clinical signs and symptoms of septic shock

Additional Antibiotic Recommendations
If fever persists without an obvious source for 72 hr or clinical deterioration occurs, consider addition of aminoglycoside or vancomycin (if not already receiving)

If perirectal infection, abdominal pain, or odontogentic focus, additional anaerobic coverage may be necessary

If fever persists for > 5 days on broad spectrum antibiotics, consider antifungal therapy

Rev 5/04

Figure 12.2 **Pennsylvania Hospital neutropenic fever pathway. (*continued*)**
Source: Provided courtesy of Pennsylvania Hospital.

	During the hospital stay	
Tests	Admission: • Chest X-ray if severe crisis chest pain or fever • Blood tests • Urine tests • Possibly other tests as determined by your doctor • EKG • Pulse oximeter	Successive days: • Blood tests
Treatments	• Temperature, pulse, blood pressure • Measure fluid taken in and put out • Pain assessed at regular intervals using 0–10 pain scale, possible oxygen	
Lines and tubes	• IV catheter or aggressive fluid by mouth	
Medications	• Possibly IV fluids • Pain medication • Stool softeners and/or laxatives • Mouth rinses	
Diet	As ordered by doctor • Drink plenty of fluids • No fresh fruits or vegetables	
Activity	• As tolerated • Incentive spirometry every 1 hour	• Aim to be out of bed 2 times a day and walk in hallways once a day (increase daily)
Teaching	• Strict hand washing • No fruits or vegetables • No flowers or plants • Anyone with a respiratory infection should not enter the room	Review/discuss process with patient regarding all care, such as pain management, medication, diet, activities, tests, etc.

Revised 5/04

Figure 12.2   **Pennsylvania Hospital neutropenic fever pathway. (*continued*)**
Source: Provided courtesy of Pennsylvania Hospital.

Day of discharge	Discharge instructions
	Discharge to Home When:
	• No fever
	• Able to tolerate fluids by mouth
	• Need less than daily transfusions (RBCs or platelets)
	• Can walk without assistance
	• Decreased pain
	Teach Patient:
	• Signs and symptoms of infection
	• When to notify MD once home
	• Once home, patient may call the Outpatient Nutrition Counseling Service at 829-3286 for additional individualized nutritional counseling
• Possibly prescriptions for home antibiotics or mouth care	**Patient Should Call Doctor if She Has:**
	A temperature of 100.5°F
	Severe shaking chills
	Shortness of breath
	Persistent bleeding (nosebleeds, easy bruising, black tarry stools, or gums bleeding)
• Resume regular diet unless noted otherwise	Pain when swallowing
	Mouth that becomes sore, tender, gums swollen, or any sores in the mouth that prevent pt from eating
	Constipation for more than 48 hours
• Continue to increase activity	Extreme weakness for more than 48 hours
	Six or more water stools (diarrhea over 24 hours)
	Nausea and vomiting for more than 24 hours
	Swelling of feet or arms

Revised 5/04

Pennsylvania
Hospital

Figure 12.2   **Pennsylvania Hospital neutropenic fever pathway. (*continued*)**
Source: Provided courtesy of Pennsylvania Hospital.

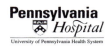

Date	Time	Nonmedication orders	(Patient Addressograph Stamp) Checked by/time

Neutropenic fever orders:

Day 1 patient care area (**Page 1 of 2**)

Date: _____ Time: _____

Attending:

Admit to:

Admitting team:

Resident: Beeper:

Intern: Beeper:

Diagnosis: Neutropenic fever

Condition:

Additional diagnosis (if any):

Allergies: ☐ No   ☐ Yes (list)

Advance directive: ☐ No   ☐ Yes

Place patient on the neutropenic fever pathway

☐ Neutropenic precautions

Activity:

☐ OOB → chair, ad lib as tolerated

☐ Bed rest bathroom privileges

☐ Neutropenic precautions

Diet:

☐ Low bacteria diet:

       No fresh fruits or vegetables, bottled or boiled water only

☐ Other: _____

Vital signs q 4 hours

Call house officer if temperature ≥ 100.5°F

☐ No fresh flowers

Medications: In computer

Heparin lock and flush q 8 hrs (must be entered in computer)

☐ Routine venous/vascular access device care

(**Continued on next page**)

Physician signature _____Beeper No. _____

Name (printed)_____

Form # 2037 A

Revised 9/2004

Not to be used for medication order

Figure 12.2   **Pennsylvania Hospital neutropenic fever pathway. (*continued*)**

Source: Provided courtesy of Pennsylvania Hospital.

Pennsylvania *Hospital*

University of Pennsylvania Health System

Date	Time	Nonmedication orders	Checked by/time
		Neutropenic fever orders:	
		Day 1 patient care area **(Page 2)**	
		If not done in ER:	
		☐ Biochemistry profile	
		☐ Culture any oral lesions for HSV × 1 (requires viral transport media)	
		☐ Stool culture for *C. difficile* toxin if diarrhea	
		☐ First dose antibiotics given after culture and prior to leaving ER	
		In am, Q day:	
		☐ CBC with differential and platelets	
		In am Q other day	
		☐ Renal, electrolyte panel	
		Consultations:	
		☐ Social worker	
		☐ Nutrition therapy	
		☐ Oncology CNS	
		Documented as done in ER:	
		☐ CBC ☐ Manual differential ☐ Platelets	
		☐ Urinalysis	
		☐ Urine C&S	
		☐ Blood cultures × 2 before antibiotics started	
		If possible: ☐ 1 peripheral ☐ 1 central line	
		☐First dose antibiotics given after culture and prior to leaving ER	
		☐ CXR	
		Physician signature _____Beeper No. _____	
		Name (printed)_____	

Form # 2037 B   **Not to be used for medication orders**
Revised 9/2004

Figure 12.2 **Pennsylvania Hospital neutropenic fever pathway. (*continued*)**
Source: Provided courtesy of Pennsylvania Hospital.

Weak, thready pulses
Tachypnea
Pale, cool, clammy skin
Anuria[1]

In **Figure 12.2**, the neutropenia pathway is initiated when a patient presents to the emergency room or is directly admitted with neutropenic fever.

REFERENCES

1. Camp-Sorrell D. Myelosuppression. In: Itano JK, Taoka KN, eds. *Core Curriculum for Oncology Nursing.* 4th ed. St. Louis, MO: Elsevier Saunders; 2005:259-274.

2. Donohue RB, Carbo G. *Abstract 121.* San Diego, CA: Oncology Nursing Society Congress; 2002.

3. National Comprehensive Cancer Network. Clinical practice guidelines in oncology v.1.2006. Myeloid Growth Factors. Available at: http://www.nccn.org/professionals/physician_gls/PDF/myeloid_growth.pdf. Accessed July 30, 2006.

4. Smith LH, Besser GS. Dietary restrictions for patients with neutropenia: a survey of institutional practices. *Oncol Nurs Forum.* 2000;27:515-520.

5. Wilson BJ. Dietary recommendations for neutropenic patients. *Semin Oncol Nurs.* 2002;18,44-49.

6. Fishbach F. A *Manual of Laborarory and Diagnostic Tests.* 6th ed. Philadelphia, PA: Lippincott; 2000.

7. National Comprehensive Cancer Network. Clinical practice guidelines in oncology. v.1.2004. Fever and Neutropenia. Available at: http://www.nccn.org/professionals/physician_gls/PDF/fever.pdf. Accessed April 20, 2005.

13

Ovarian Cancer Case Study

ML is a 66-year-old female newly diagnosed with stage 3B epithelial ovarian cancer. She reports the presence of fatigue, shortness of breath, early satiety, constipation, bloating, and a 10-pound weight gain. She states that these symptoms have gotten progressively worse in the last 6 months. ML first presented to her family doctor who, in turn, sent her to a gastroenterologist. When the GI workup proved to be negative, ML was sent to her gynecologist. A pelvic exam revealed an increase in the size and shape of her right ovary. The gynecologist felt a fluid wave and thought her weight gain was due to the presence of ascites. A transvaginal ultrasound confirmed a right ovarian mass. She was then referred to a GYN oncologist. ML was then scheduled for an exploratory laparotomy to obtain a tissue sample of the mass. The pathology results confirmed ovarian cancer. ML is now scheduled for a total abdominal hysterectomy, bilateral salpingo-oophorectomy, peritoneal cytology, omentectomy, and lymph node dissection. ML reports that she is feeling anxious about the upcoming surgery. She states that she is angry that no one paid attention to her symptoms for 6 months. She has been married for 46 years, has no children, and is a homemaker. ML was diagnosed with early stage breast cancer 10 years ago and was successfully treated with lumpectomy and radiation at that time. Family history is significant in that ML has a mother and sister who were diagnosed with breast cancer and another sister who died of ovarian cancer.

What function do the ovaries have?

The ovaries produce and release ova, estrogen progesterone, and testosterone.[1]

What risk factors does ML have for developing ovarian cancer?

Age, nulliparity, and family history of breast and ovarian cancer are ML's risk factors. The peak incidence of occurrence of ovarian cancer occurs from 60-64 years. Both nulliparity and infertility place a woman at increased risk. ML has both a personal and family history of cancer. A personal or family history of breast, endometrial, or colon cancer is important to assess.[1] The most important risk factor for ovarian cancer is a family history with a first-degree relative such as a mother, daughter, or sister. The highest risk appears to be 2 or more first-degree relatives with ovarian cancer. The risk is less for women with 1 first-degree relative and 1 second-degree relative such as a grandmother or aunt with ovarian cancer. About 10% of epithelial ovarian cancers are familial.[1-2]

Is ovarian cancer a common cancer in women?

No, ovarian cancer accounts for only 3% of cancers in women. There will be an estimated 20,180 new cases and 15,000 women will die of ovarian cancer in 2006. Ovarian cancer causes more deaths than any other cancer of the female reproductive system. It is the second most common gynecologic cancer following cancer of the uterine corpus.[3]

Can ovarian cancer be detected early?

Ovarian cancer is difficult to detect early because no accurate screening test is currently available. Pelvic exam, as seen in ML's case, can occasionally detect ovarian cancer, but generally not until the cancer is at an advanced stage. This is because the ovaries are usually physically inaccessible. Women who are at increased risk should be offered a thorough pelvic exam, a transvaginal ultrasound, and a blood test for the tumor marker CA125. Increased vigilance in high-risk individuals could lead to earlier diagnosis.[3]

Why is it important for a gynecological surgical oncologist to do the surgery?

Studies suggest that women who have advanced disease have a more successful outcome when this type of specialist is involved. This is because the ovarian cancer can then be accurately staged and treated.[3]

What should the nurse teach ML about her upcoming surgery?

She should teach ML coughing, turning, deep breathing, splinting, and incentive spirometry. She should review what the postoperative schedule for these activities will be and review how to use the incentive spirometer. The nurse should ask ML for a return demonstration. She should teach ML that early ambulation will promote a smooth recovery. She should show her where her incision will be and describe any tubes and drains that will be present postoperatively. The plan for postoperative pain management should be outlined. ML should be informed where to report the morning of surgery, as well as where her family should wait during the surgery and how news will be communicated with family.[4]

The morning after surgery is performed the surgeon tells ML that all visible tumor is removed. Biopsy of the bladder, liver, diaphragm, and appendix are all negative. She recovers well from her surgery. ML is scheduled for 3 cycles of paclitaxel (Taxol) and carboplatin (Paraplatin). If ML has a good clinical response she will be scheduled for a second-look restaging laparotomy.

Why is a second-look surgery planned?

The goal of the procedure is to detect any residual tumor, debulk any remaining tumor, and determine future chemotherapy treatment. If ML responds to chemotherapy, at least 3 more cycles will be given.[1]

What teaching should the nurse do before ML begins chemotherapy?

The nurse begins with paclitaxel. She tells ML that this drug will be given intravenously every 3 weeks over about 3 hours. She should teach ML that she will be given medications before the paclitaxel infusion to help prevent nausea and to help prevent allergic reaction. She should teach her that common side effects include hair loss and a low blood count, which means that ML is at increased risk of infection, allergic reaction, numbness and tingling in her hands and feet beginning with fingers and toes, and achy muscles and joints. Less common side effects include mouth sores, diarrhea, nausea and vomiting, low blood pressure, and slowing of the heart rate. She should tell ML that carboplatin will be administered by vein following the paclitaxel infusion over about 30 minutes. Carboplatin also lowers the white blood cell count. In addition, it lowers the platelet count, which places ML at increased risk for bleeding. High doses can affect kidney function; other side effects include nausea, vomiting, fatigue, decreased appetite, diarrhea, constipation, taste changes, numbness and tingling in the hands and feet, beginning with fingers and toes, ringing in the ears, and burning with urination. This drug can cause an allergic reaction after several doses. Discharge instructions should include instructing the patient to report fever greater than 100.5°F, chills, cough, shortness of breath, sore throat, difficulty seeing, nausea, vomiting, constipation or diarrhea that is not relieved by medication and lasts more than 24-48 hours, unusual bleeding or bruising, lower back or side pain, difficulty or pain when urinating, numbness and tingling in fingers or toes, and redness or tenderness at the IV site. The nurse should give ML a tour of the treatment area. ML should be encouraged to bring snacks or lunch if she will be receiving treatment at mealtime. She should bring items that will help her to be comfortable, such as reading materials or music. All verbal instructions should be reinforced with written materials.[5]

What route other than the intravenous route is used to deliver chemotherapy to ovarian cancer patients?

The intraperitoneal route is also used to deliver chemotherapy. The advantages of intraperitoneal chemotherapy are that higher concentrations of drugs are delivered to the tumor with less systemic side effects. The National Cancer Institute now recommends that women with advanced disease who successfully undergo surgery receive a combination of intraperitoneal and intravenous chemotherapy.[6]

What is ascites?

Ascites is an abnormal accumulation of fluid in the abdominal cavity that is not reabsorbed into the systemic circulation. In ML's case, it is due to the ovarian cancer. Ascites occurs in 30%-54% of patients with ovarian cancer. Malignant ascites accounts for 10% of all cases of ascites, most of them are intra-abdominal malignancies or liver metastasis. Extra-abdominal cancers include breast, lung, lymphatic, colon, gastric, pancreatic, mesothelioma, testicular, and sarcoma cancers.[7]

What does ascites mean as far as ML's prognosis is concerned?

Ascites is not associated with a favorable prognosis. Factors that are associated with the most favorable prognosis include younger age, good performance status, cell type other than mucinous or clear, lower stage, well-differentiated tumor, smaller disease volume prior to any surgical debulking, absence of ascites, and smaller residual tumor following primary cytoreductive surgery.[2]

What are some ways the nurse can assess for the presence of ascites?

She can weigh ML and note the amount of weight gain if she has gained weight, along with the presence or absence of abdominal distention. She can measure abdominal girth and look for everted umbilicus, stretched skin, bulging flanks, and lower extremity edema. Finally, she can check for fluid wave.[7]

How is ascites treated?

The best treatment of malignant ascites is to treat the underlying cause. ML will receive chemotherapy to treat the ovarian cancer, which will, in turn, have an effect on her ascites. Noncancer causes need to be ruled out. Repeated paracentesis removal of ascites fluid leads to protein depletion. Peritoneovenous shunts divert fluid from the abdomen into the blood circulation. LeVeen and Denver shunts are most frequently used. Shunting malignant fluid causes cancer cells to travel through the circulation. External drains used to remove ascites fluid have a 43% incidence of infection. Some new approaches utilizing intracavity therapy are being studied. Fluid and dietary restrictions are only helpful when the patient has cirrhosis.[7]

What are some psychological issues that ML may face?

ML will be coping with a new diagnosis of cancer. She is also dealing with an advanced stage cancer. Diagnosis is often delayed because no good screening tools exist. Many women deal with the possibility that their ovarian cancer may not be curable but is in fact a chronic illness. We have a hint that ML is having difficulty dealing with her diagnosis because she is verbalizing anger that her symptoms were not addressed earlier.[1]

How can ML's nurse help ML to address these issues?

The nurse can suggest that ML attend an ovarian cancer support group. The American Cancer Society has a list of local area support groups. In addition, several ovarian cancer advocacy groups exist. ML may want to participate in 1-on-1 counseling with a psychologist or participate in another form of counseling, such as art therapy or music therapy.[1] A list of ovarian cancer resources is found in **Table 13.1**.

Table 13.1   **Ovarian Cancer Resources**

Conversations!
www.ovarian-news.com
The International Newsletter for Those Fighting Ovarian Cancer

Gilda's Club
www.gildasclub.org
Free of charge and not-for-profit, Gilda's Club offers support and networking groups, lectures, workshops, and social events in a nonresidential, home-like setting.

National Ovarian Cancer Coalition
www.ovarian.org
Its mission is to raise awareness about ovarian cancer and to promote education about this disease. By dispelling myths and misunderstandings, the coalition is committed to improving the overall survival rate and quality of life for women with ovarian cancer.

Ovarian Cancer National Alliance
www.ovariancancer.org
Its mission is to conquer ovarian cancer by uniting individuals and organizations in a national movement.

REFERENCES

1. Temple SV, Umstead CH. Nursing care of the client with cancers of the reproductive system. In: Itano JK, Taoka KN, eds. *Core Curriculum for Oncology Nursing*. 4th ed. St. Louis, MO: Elsevier Saunders; 2005:566-570.

2. National Cancer Institute. Ovarian epithelial cancer (PDQ): treatment. Available at: http://www.nci.nih.gov/cancertopics/pdq/treatment/ovarianepithelial/healthprofessional. Accessed February 28, 2006.

3. American Cancer Society. Cancer Facts and Figures 2006. Atlanta, GA: Author; 2006.

4. Szopa TJ. Nursing implications of surgical treatment. In: Itano JK, Taoka JK, eds. *Core Curriculum for Oncology Nursing*. 4th ed. St. Louis, MO: Elsevier Saunders; 2005:736-747.

5. Wilkes GM, Barton-Burke M. *Oncology Nursing Drug Handbook*. Sudbury, MA: Jones and Bartlett Publishers; 2005:86-89, 238-245.

6. Abeloff MD, ed. NCI urges IV/IP chemo for advanced ovarian cancer. *Oncology News International*. 2006;15(2):1.

7. Berendt M, D'Agostino S. Alterations in nutrition. In: Itano JK, Taoka KN, eds. *Core Curriculum for Oncology Nursing*. 4th ed. St. Louis, MO: Elsevier Saunders; 2005:312-315.

14

Pain Case Study

JB is a 79-year-old male diagnosed with multiple myeloma involving the bone including the spine 6 months ago. He complains of severe, sharp, throbbing back pain which also started 6 months ago and has progressively worsened over the last several months. JB describes the pain as most severe when he wakes up. He rates it as 9 on a 0-10 pain scale. He is currently taking 1-2 oxycodone with acetaminophen (Percocet) every 4 hours as needed. Following 2 oxycodone with acetaminophen, the pain goes down to a 4, which JB says is an acceptable level of pain to him. He reports taking 2 oxycodone with acetaminophen on average 4 times a day since diagnosis. He takes a dose before bedtime but none during the night. He is concerned about the amount of pain pills he is taking and tells his nurse that he is afraid of becoming addicted to them.

What criteria are used to measure pain?

First and foremost, believe the patient's report of pain. Over 30 years ago, pain expert Margo McCaffery first said, "Pain is whatever the patient says it is, existing whenever they say it does."[1]

Important Criteria to Keep in Mind

Location: where are all the pain sites?

Characteristics (words to describe the pain)

Possible neuropathic pain characteristics: sharp, stabbing, shooting, and burning.

Possible nociceptive pain includes both somatic and visceral pain. Characteristics: throbbing, dull, aching, and crampy.

Duration: Is it constant or intermittent? When does it start? Are there good days and bad days?

Assess aggravating and relieving factors: Pain with movement? Relief with rest? Pain constant? Pain unprovoked?[2]

Intensity: In adults, the 0-10 numeric pain scale (**Figure 14.1**) is used most often.[3]

Is JB's pain acute or chronic? Explain the difference.

JB's pain is chronic because it has lasted for more than 3 months. Acute pain is defined as pain that lasts for a short period of time, usually less than 6 months, is due to a known acute event, and disappears after the event is resolved. Chronic pain is defined as persistent pain lasting for long periods of time. Cancer pain includes both acute and chronic pain. Both acute and chronic cancer pain can be

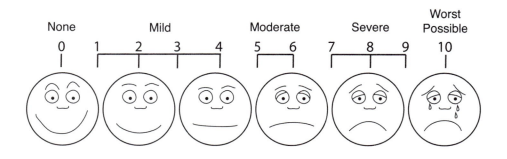

Figure 14.1　**Numeric pain scale.**
Source: Copyright Supportive Oncology Services, 2005.

from treatment, for example postmastectomy pain, radiation-induced mucositis, or chemotherapy related neuropathy or from the cancer itself.[4]

Is JB's pain visceral, somatic, or neuropathic?

JB's pain is somatic.

Why is JB's pain classified as somatic?

Somatic pain is defined as damage to skin, blood vessels, subcutaneous tissue, fascia, and muscle. It is well localized, worse with movement. It is treated with NSAIDs and opioids. Patients describe somatic pain as aching, squeezing, stabbing, or throbbing. Arthritis and bone pain related to cancer are 2 common examples of somatic pain. The most common somatic pain description is an aching pain that is exacerbated by movement or weight bearing. Visceral pain is defined as organ (viscera) damage. It is diffuse, poorly localized, and may need high doses of opioids to obtain relief. NSAIDs may be added to the regimen. Visceral pain is associated with obstruction, perforation, and distention of hollow organs. Both somatic and visceral pain are known as nociceptive because they occur as a result of stimulation of pain fibers (nociceptors) in deep or cutaneous tissue. Neuropathic pain is defined as nerve damage, burning, painful numbness, tingling. It is not affected by movement and is treated with anticonvulsants, e.g., gabapentin (Neurontin), and/or antidepressants, e.g., amitriptyline (Elavil). The patient will use words like numbness, tingling, shooting, burning, stabbing, and sharp to describe his pain. Peripheral neuropathic pain is caused by injury along the peripheral nerves; this is the type of pain that the patient describes as numbness and tingling. Centrally mediated pain is described as radiating and shooting and may include burning and aching.[2,4,5]

Is JB's amount of pain relief with the oxycodone with acetaminophen acceptable?

No, it is unacceptable.

Why isn't the amount of pain relief acceptable?

Although JB reports adequate relief with oxycodone with acetaminophen after he takes it, he is not taking it around the clock and wakes up in pain. Around-the-clock dosing is recommended for chronic pain. A long-acting regimen should be put into place with a breakthrough medication available prn.[6]

What is one way that JB's pain regimen might be changed?

A long-acting medication could be used instead of oxycodone with acetaminophen. One of the tablets JB takes contains 5 mg oxycodone and 325 mg acetaminophen. JB is using 2 tablets approximately 4 times a day, which is 8 tablets a day. This is the equivalent of 40 mg oxycodone and 2600 mg acetaminophen. There is a maximum dose ceiling of acetaminophen, which is 4 grams. JB cannot take more than that amount per day. Sustained release oxycodone (OxyContin) is a long-acting narcotic analgesic. Sustained release oxycodone comes in 10 mg, 20 mg, 40 mg and 80 mg tablets. JB could take a 20 mg sustained release oxycodone tablet every 12 hours with 2 tablets of oxycodone with acetaminophen every 4 hours as needed. This would give JB equianalgesic and more consistent relief, and if needed his dose could be increased based on how much prn breakthrough medication he is taking. Breakthrough doses are usually calculated as 10% of the daily dose and given every 2-4 hours as needed.[6]

What are the side effects of narcotic analgesics and how could they be addressed?

Narcotic analgesics reduce smooth muscle motility. This means that JB may experience constipation. JB should be assessed for usual bowel habits. The nurse should instruct JB to increase fluid and fiber intake. A stimulating laxative, not just a stool softener, is usually necessary because of the reduction in bowel motility. Other side effects include nausea and vomiting, somnolence, urinary retention, dizziness, confusion, rashes, and itching. Most patients will develop tolerance to all of these symptoms, except constipation, in about 3 to 5 days. Antiemetics are used for nausea and vomiting and antihistamines are used for itching.[6]

How should the nurse address JB's concern about becoming addicted to pain medication?

This is a common concern for patients with cancer. Very few people taking narcotic analgesics develop a problem with addiction. If a patient has been taking a narcotic for a long period of time, his body will become accustomed to it and will react if the medication is stopped abruptly. This means that the body develops a physical dependence on the medication. Narcotic analgesics should be tapered over a period of time, allowing the body to adjust to a lower level of the medicine, and not stopped abruptly. The body can also develop a tolerance for a pain medication. This means that over time, pain will not be relieved by the same dose of medication. A higher dose will be needed. Development of tolerance to a drug does not indicate that a person is becoming addicted to a drug. Addiction involves a strong psychological dependence on a drug. People who are addicted take a drug to satisfy an emotional need and have no control over taking the drug. They continue to use the drug even if they are harming themselves.[7]

What is one factor to consider related to starting a narcotic analgesic in a person of JB's age?

Older patients experience the same amounts of pain that younger patients do but the adage "start low and go slow" is important to remember because older patients may have reduced renal and hepatic function. Medications may remain longer in an older person's system.[8]

What are 3 common barriers to pain management that cancer patients experience?

Some common barriers include inexperience and lack of education on the part of the health care providers, fear of addiction on the part of the patient, family or health care providers, and fear that pain will be not able to be controlled as the end of life approaches if pain medicine is used before then.[3]

JB wants to try an integrative pain management modality along with his medication management. He asks what is available to him. What can the nurse tell him?

There are many effective integrative therapies that can be used along with the pain medications such as acupuncture, Shiatsu massage, music therapy, art therapy, Reiki, and distraction activities like watching funny movies or visiting with friends. Like the name integrative suggests, these therapies are used along with, not instead of, conventional therapies.[9]

REFERENCES

1. McCaffrey M. Pain management: Problems and progress. In: McCaffrey M, Pasero C, eds. *Pain: Clinical Manual*. 2nd ed. St. Louis, MO: Mosby; 1999:5.

2. Pasero C, Paice JA, McCaffery M. Basic mechanisms underlying the causes and effects of pain. In: McCaffrey M, Pasero C, eds. *Pain: Clinical Manual*. 2nd ed. St. Louis, MO: Mosby; 1999:15-31.

3. McCaffrey M, Pasero C. Underlying complexities, misconceptions, and practical tools. In: McCaffrey M, Pasero C, eds. *Pain: Clinical Manual*. 2nd ed. St. Louis, MO: Mosby; 1999:35-99.

4. Brant JM. Comfort. In: Itano JK, Taoka KN, eds. *Core Curriculum for Oncology Nursing*. 4th ed. St. Louis, MO: Elsevier Saunders; 2005:3-15.

5. National Comprehensive Cancer Network. Clinical practice guidelines in oncology v.2.2005. Adult Cancer Pain. Available at: http://www.nccn.org/professionals/physician_gls/PDF/pain.pdf. Accessed July 20, 2005.

6. Pasero C, Portenoy RK, McCaffery, M. Opioid analgesics. In: McCaffrey M, Pasero C, eds. *Pain: Clinical Manual*. 2nd ed. St. Louis, MO: Mosby; 1999:161-299.

7. Compton P. Substance abuse. In: McCaffrey M, Pasero C, eds. *Pain: Clinical Manual*. 2nd ed. St. Louis, MO: Mosby; 1999:428-462.

8. Pasero C, Reed BA, McMaffery M. Pain in the elderly. In: McCaffrey M, Pasero C, eds. *Pain: Clinical Manual*. 2nd ed. St. Louis, MO: Mosby; 1999:674-706.

9. McCaffrey M, Pasero C. Nondrug approaches to pain. In: McCaffrey M, Pasero C, eds. *Pain: Clinical Manual*. 2nd ed. St. Louis, MO: Mosby; 1999:399-421.

15

Chemotherapy-Related Peripheral Neuropathy Case Study

MA is a 42-year-old female diagnosed with stage II-B ductal breast cancer 4 months ago. She is receiving dose-dense chemotherapy with doxorubicin (Adriamycin) and cyclophosphamide (Cytoxan) every 2 weeks followed by paclitaxel (Taxol) every 2 weeks. She arrives at the clinic for her last dose of paclitaxel. During the assessment she tells her nurse that she is experiencing moderate numbness and tingling in her fingers and on the bottoms of her feet, starting with her toes. MA's nurse reviews her nursing assessment from the last visit and sees that MA complained of some mild numbness and tingling in the same areas. Past medical history includes adult onset diabetes.

What is peripheral neuropathy?

Neuropathy is defined as inflammation, injury, or degeneration of the peripheral nerve fibers.[1] Usually it is related to damage of the nerve filaments in the nerve axon.

What should be assessed related to peripheral neuropathy prior to the first dose of chemotherapy?

It is important to assess for preexisting conditions that can cause neuropathy in order to establish a baseline. For example, MA has diabetes. Other conditions that can cause neuropathy include alcoholism, vitamin B_{12} deficiency, arthrosclerosis, ataxia, and thyroid dysfunction. Previous cancer treatment can be a cause of preexisting neuropathy (see **Table 15.1**).[1-3]

What chemotherapeutic agent in MA's regimen can cause peripheral neuropathy?

Paclitaxel is associated with a 60% incidence of any symptoms of neuropathy. Other chemotherapeutic agents, interferon, and radiation can all cause neuropathy.[2] Paclitaxel affects the sensory nervous system and usually manifests itself in the form of numbness and tingling in the extremities. The autonomic and motor nervous systems can also be affected at higher doses.[4]

List 3 different types of chemotherapy-related peripheral neuropathy.

Symptoms will vary depending on which part of the nervous system is being affected.

Autonomic Nervous System
BP (orthostatic hypotension)
Intestinal mobility (constipation or ileus)

Sensory Nervous System
Large fiber vibration and proprioception (sense of position, movement, and force)

Motor Nervous System
Reflexes
Strength[1-3]

Table 15.1   Chemotherapy Agents Likely to Cause Neurotoxicity

High incidence (very common, > 80% incidence)

Cisplatin	Interferon (especially at HD)
Interleukin-1 (if patient develops capillary leak syndrome)	

Moderate incidence (common, 20%-80% incidence)

Arsenic trioxide	Methotrexate (IT, HD)
Carmustine (intra-arterial)	Oxaliplatin, ormaplatin
Cytosine arabinoside (HD)	Paclitaxel
Docetaxel	Procarbazine
Hexamethylmelamine	Suramin
Ifosfamide	Tretinoin
1-asparaginase	Vincristine, vinblastine, vinorelbine

Uncommon (20% incidence)

Busulfan	Fludarabine
Capecitabine	5-fluorouracil
Cladribine	Pentostatin
Etoposide	Teniposide

IT = intrathecal HD = high dose

Source: Chemotherapeutic agents that induce peripheral neuropathy. In: Wilkes GM, Barton-Burke M. *2005 Oncology Nursing Drug Handbook.* Sudbury, MA: Jones and Bartlett; 381, based on data from Armstrong T, Rust D, Kohtz JR (1997); Cheson BD, Vena DA, Foss FM, Sorensen JM (1994); Furlong TG (1993); Weiss RB (2001).

What is the pattern of distribution for chemotherapy-related peripheral neuropathy?

The nurse can expect a "stocking-glove" distribution. This means that the neuropathy starts in the tips of the fingers and toes and moves upwards as was seen in MA's case.[1,3]

How should MA's nurse perform an assessment related to peripheral neuropathy?

The nurse should begin by asking MA about the presence, location, severity, characteristics, and aggravating and relieving factors of pain as well as the presence of numbness and tingling. Patients often do not associate numbness and tingling with pain, so asking about both is necessary. The nurse should check for changes in sensation. This can be achieved by testing the extremities for pain or light touch sensation when the patient's eyes are closed. She should assess for changes in motor function. Can MA button her shirt or tie her shoes? Is she having any other changes in her activities of daily living (ADLs)? Is there a change in gait, hesitation, unsteadiness, or foot drop? Finally, her nurse should assess for changes in bowel function. Patients experiencing autonomic nervous system neuropathy could have constipation or paralytic ileus.[1,3] **Table 15.2** is a useful grading criteria that can help nurses accurately describe the severity of neuropathy.

How is chemotherapy-related neuropathy managed?

Pharmacologic and nonpharmacologic interventions can be used. Pharmacologic management includes anticonvulsants such as gabapentim (Neurontin), tricyclic antidepressants, opioids, and transdermal agents such as the lidocaine patch.[5] Nonpharmacologic management includes exercise, massage, acupuncture, and hydrotherapy. PT and OT can be very helpful with assistive devices and strength exercises.[1,3]

Should MA's last dose of paclitaxel be withheld?

No, it is important for MA to receive the planned dose of chemotherapy on time. To not do so would negate the survival benefit obtained from adjuvant chemotherapy.

What safety measures should MA be taught?

MA should be instructed to remove slippery throw rugs or bath mats and replace them with nonskid ones, make sure her home is well lit, turn down the water

Table 15.2 **National Cancer Institute Common Toxicity Criteria: Neuropathy**

	Grade				
Toxicity	**0**	**1**	**2**	**3**	**4**
Neuropathy-motor	Normal	Subjective weakness but no objective findings	Mild objective weakness interfering with function, but not interfering with activities of daily living	Objective weakness interfering with activities of daily living	Paralysis
Neuropathy-sensory	Normal	Loss of deep tendon reflexes of paresthesia (including tingling), but not interfering with function	Objective sensory loss or paresthesia (including tingling), interfering with function, but not interfering with activities of daily living	Sensory loss or paresthesia interfering with activities of daily living	Permanent sensory loss that interferes with function

Source: Wilkes GM, Barton-Burke M. *2005 Oncology Nursing Drug Handbook.* Sudbury, MA: Jones and Bartlett; 2005:1034-1035.

temperature to avoid burns, add a shower chair and hand railing in the bathroom, use liquid dispensed soap instead of bar soap, wear cotton socks and well fitting shoes, use rubber gloves when washing dishes, and, in general, be aware of decreased sensation.[1]

References

1. Almadrones LA, Arcot R. Patient guide to peripheral neuropathy. *Oncol Nurs Forum*. 1999;26(8):1359-1362.

2. Sweeney CW. Understanding peripheral neuropathy in patients with cancer: background and patient assessment. *Clin J Oncol Nurs*. 2002;6:163-166.

3. Armstrone T, Amadrones LA, Gilbert MR. Chemotherapy induced peripheral neuropathy. *Oncol Nurs Forum*. 2005;32(2):305-311.

4. Paclitaxel [package insert]. Princeton, NJ; Bristol Myers Squibb Company; March, 2003.

5. Lidoderm Lidocaine Patch 5% [package insert]. Chadds Ford, PA; Endo Pharmaceuticals; August, 2006.

16

Lung Cancer with
Pleural Effusion Case Study

MJ is a 63-year-old male admitted to the unit with dyspnea and a productive cough. He says he has had these symptoms for over a month and just started to spike a temperature yesterday. MJ says he has been feeling fatigued lately and has had some chest discomfort from excessive coughing.

Upon assessment, the nurse finds that MJ has a temperature of 102°F, his pulse is 84, and his respirations are at 24. He has a productive cough and is bringing up yellow/green sputum. He is complaining of chest discomfort from coughing. MJ has bilateral rales in both lung fields. He states he was a 2-packs-per-day smoker but recently quit. He denies any hemoptysis. He states he has recently lost about 15 pounds.

A diagnostic workup is started on MJ to determine the cause of his fever and cough. The physician orders the following tests and treatments:

Chest X-ray
Sputum for cytology
Pulmonary function tests
CBC, SMA10

IV fluid of 1 L d5 1/2 NSS at 100 cc/hour
Cefepime (Maxipime) 1 gram IV q 12 hours

MJ asks why these tests are ordered. What should the nurse tell him?

The nurse should explain that these tests are being ordered to find the cause of his fever and cough. The chest X-ray will produce an image of the internal structures of the chest to locate any abnormality that may be present. Sputum cytology is a microscopic exam of the sputum that identifies cellular abnormalities that do not show up on a chest X-ray. Blood work is ordered to check for infection and to make sure the blood counts are not abnormal. Pulmonary function tests are done to assess current lung function to ascertain how well he could function with limited lung capacity if surgery becomes necessary. The IV fluids are to prevent dehydration and the antibiotic is to help reduce the fever, assuming the cause is pneumonia.[1]

The chest X-ray shows a shadow in the left upper lobe that looks like a tumor. The sputum cytology comes back inconclusive. The physician orders a low-dose helical CT scan of the chest, PET scan, and a bronchoscopy with biopsy.

Why are these tests ordered in addition to the ones listed previously?

Diagnostic workup can include chest X-ray, sputum cytology, bronchoscopy with biopsy, video-assisted thoracoscopy, ultrasound-guided fine-needle aspiration, CT, PET, and MRI. Newer tools, including low-dose helical CT scans and PET scans, can detect lung cancer earlier and when tumors are smaller than conventional X-rays can. These advances will allow more patients to become surgical candidates. Lung cancer cannot be definitively diagnosed without a cytology or biopsy specimen, which is examined in the pathology department. The CT scan is being ordered to further evaluate the tumor that showed up on the chest X-ray. It will also further determine the size and location of the tumor as well as any metastasis to the lymph nodes in the surrounding area. When lung cancer has spread, some of the first areas it goes to are the lymph nodes and abdominal area. The bronchoscopy is ordered to look for additional tumors and to obtain a tissue sample to determine the staging of the disease so a treatment course can be developed. A PET scan is done to evaluate mediastinal lymph node involvement and to look for metastasis elsewhere.[1]

The pathology report, along with the diagnostic workup, confirms that MJ has a stage 2 non-small cell lung cancer (NSCLC).

What does this mean?

There are 2 basic types of lung cancer: small cell lung cancer (SCLC) and non-small cell lung cancer (NSCLC). Treatment varies according to type of lung cancer, so it is important to differentiate the 2. NSCLC is the most amenable to surgery.

NSCLC is comprised of 3 subgroups, which are named for the type of lung cancer cells found in each group. In the first group, adenocarcinoma is the most common of all lung cancers, making up almost half of total cases. It grows along the outer edges of the lungs and tissue lining the bronchi. It is the most common lung cancer in women. It is associated with a high likelihood of metastasis.

Epidermoid carcinoma is also known as squamous cell carcinoma. It begins in a central location in the lungs, such as the bronchi, and may remain longer in the lungs without spreading than other types of lung cancer. Many patients with epidermoid lung cancer are surgical candidates. This type of lung cancer is easier to resect because of its location. It is associated with a better prognosis.

Large cell lung carcinoma is found in the smaller bronchi. It is more difficult to resect and is associated with a poor prognosis.[2]

What is the difference between SCLC and NSCLC?

SCLC (oat cell cancer) is a more aggressive disease and is less common than NSCLC. The majority of small cell lung cancer is associated with smoking tobacco. It arises from a different cellular linage than NSCLC. It usually starts in the bronchi. It is characterized by rapidly growing cells and early spread to other organs. Small cell lung cancer is more sensitive to chemotherapy than NSCLC.

Because SCLC is considered a systemic disease on diagnosis, surgery is done less often.[2]

Accurate classification and staging are extremely important in defining treatment options for patients with lung cancer. This process has an impact on quality of life. Appropriate treatment is either curative or palliative. If a lung cancer is inadequately staged, a patient might undergo unnecessary treatment, including surgery. They might sacrifice precious quality time with family and friends due to difficult side effects. Staging for NSCLC follows the American Joint Commission on Cancer (AJCC) TNM system. T divides lung cancer into 8 numerical stages. It classifies and divides the primary tumor into categories based on size, location, and invasiveness. N divides it into categories representing regional lymph node status. M indicates the presence or absence of distant metastasis.[3]

Stage 2 NSCLC indicates that the cancer is in 1 lung and has invaded local lymph nodes. MJ's pathology reveals that the cell type is adenocarcinoma.

What are the treatment options for MJ?

Based on the diagnostic workup, treatment options for MJ are surgery alone, radiation therapy alone, and a combination of surgery and radiation therapy with or without chemotherapy.

Surgical options for lung cancer include lobectomy, which is generally indicated for smaller tumors, pneumonectomy, and wedge resection. Treatment options depend on a variety of factors that include the type of lung cancer, location of the tumor, and spread to adjoining structures. In addition, the overall health and performance status of the patient helps to determine the various treatment options available.[1]

MJ asks for explanations about the different surgical options that his physician reviewed with him. What should he be told?

A lobectomy removes the entire lobe of the lung. A pneumonectomy removes the whole lung. A wedge resection removes part of the lung and some surrounding tissue.[1]

MJ and his physician opt for surgery followed by chemotherapy. The physician feels that MJ is a good candidate for surgery based on his history and the location of his tumor. He recommends a wedge resection using video-assisted thoracic surgery (VATS). Video-assisted thoracic surgery (VATS) is a newer surgical technique that can be used diagnostically with video-assisted thoracoscopy or therapeutically with video-assisted thoracotomy for early-stage disease. Small thoracotomy incisions are made, and thoracoscopic instruments are inserted through the incisions. The surgeon can then visualize the chest and mediastinum on a monitor. VATS works best when used for small peripheral nodules. VATS involves 1 to 4 small incisions and can be used for excision of lung lesions, biopsy of mediastinal masses, wedge resection of tumors, and other exploratory procedures. Because VATS involves less invasive surgery, it is associated with less postoperative discomfort, less need for postoperative analgesia due to less dissection and spreading of ribs, shorter recovery, and decreased length of stay.[4]

What should the nurse teach MJ and his family about his preoperative and postoperative care?

Thoracic surgery has a high risk of complications. Candidates are carefully selected to determine if they are able to withstand surgery. Cardiopulmonary status is carefully evaluated. Nurses involved in the preoperative care of lung-cancer patients are essential in facilitating a successful recovery. They should evaluate MJ's ability to use an incentive spirometer, cough, turn, deep breathe, splint, and perform upper and lower extremity range-of-motion exercises postoperatively. They should teach him these activities preoperatively with a return postoperative demonstration. They should teach MJ and his family about what he will experience before, during, and after surgery and instruct MJ that he may have nothing by mouth after midnight before surgery. MJ is most likely going to the intensive care unit (ICU) postoperatively. A tour and discussion about the ICU, monitoring devices, and ventilator can reduce postoperative anxiety, as MJ and his family are then prepared for the experience. MJ should expect to spend 24-48 hours in a monitored setting. In addition to the ventilator, he should be prepared to expect that he might have chest tubes, compression stockings, a

Foley catheter, and intravenous fluids. His family should know where to wait and how information will be communicated. Patients who smoke should be strongly encouraged to quit smoking and given information about smoking cessation options.[1] The nurse should teach MJ that he is a part of a multidisciplinary team, which includes the physician, nurse, social worker, dietitian, physical therapist, chaplain, and other practitioners who give supportive care. The nurse should monitor MJ's vital signs per his institution's policy and procedure for postoperative patients. They should be monitored every 4 hours for the first 24 hours. He should assess MJ's pain frequently using the 0-10 pain scale and document accordingly. MJ should be out of bed his first postoperative night and be ambulated as soon as possible to prevent postoperative complications such as pneumonia and deep vein thrombosis. He should cough, turn, and deep breathe frequently and use his incentive spirometer 10 times an hour. The nurse assesses MJ's incision and monitors his chest tube for drainage. He should monitor intake and output every 4 hours. MJ should void within 8 hours of surgery. The nurse would closely monitor MJ's IV fluids as well.[1]

MJ has an uneventful postoperative course and is discharged home with his wife and children. His plan of care includes postoperative radiation therapy after he has healed.

MJ asks why he will have radiation therapy. What should the nurse tell him?

He should tell him that even though the surgeon feels that he got all the cancer, there may be some residual cells that have been left behind. Radiation therapy is for local control of the cancer. Having radiation therapy will help to eliminate any leftover cancer cells.[1]

MJ does well for about a year, and then he presents to the unit with dyspnea, cough, oxygen saturation of 88%, and chest pain. He is also tachycardic with decreased breath sounds on the left side. A cardiac problem is ruled out. A chest X-ray shows a left pleural effusion.

What is a pleural effusion?

It is an abnormal fluid collection in the pleural space. It is usually due to heart failure, surgery, or a malignancy. The pleural space contains 5 to 15 ml of fluid, which prevents friction when the pleural surfaces move. More than 25 ml is considered an effusion, although up to 300 ml may accumulate before symptoms appear. The drainage will vary depending upon the cause of the effusion.[5]

Based on MJ's history, the pleural effusion is probably related to recurrence of the lung cancer.

What is the next course of action?

MJ needs to have a chest tube inserted. The nurse will need to be available to assist with the procedure and support MJ. The insertion can be done in the operating room, in radiology, or at the bedside. This is a painful procedure so the nurse would have to assure that MJ has adequate pain medication and a local anesthetic is given prior to the chest tube insertion.

Why does MJ have a chest tube inserted?

He has the chest tube (also known as a thoracostomy tube or thoracic catheter) inserted to remove the malignant fluid from the pleural space. A chest tube is commonly inserted to resolve pneumothorax, hemothorax, or pleural effusion or to drain blood from the mediastinum after open-heart surgery.[6]

What 3 nursing diagnoses are most appropriate for MJ?

The following diagnoses are key:

1. Knowledge deficit related to the recurrence of lung cancer diagnosis and impending course of treatment
2. Altered respiratory status related to his pleural effusion and chest tube drainage system
3. Pain R/T his disease progression and symptoms

The goal of treatment for a pleural effusion is to relieve the patient's pain, dyspnea, and respiratory compromise; treat the underlying cause of the effusion; and prevent fluid from reaccumulating in the lung.[6]

What nursing interventions should the nurse provide for this patient?

He should assess MJ's cardiopulmonary status at least every 4 hours and check the chest tube insertion site every 4 hours for inflammation, drainage from the site, signs of infection, or subcutaneous emphysema. He should check the dressings at the chest tube site and change them according to hospital policy.[6]

The nurse should encourage coughing, turning, and deep breathing every 2 hours to promote lung expansion and prevent atelectasis. He should encourage ambulation. MJ's chest tube needs to be monitored every 4 hours; the nurse should check the tube for patency and kinks and record the amount and color of pleural drainage.[6]

What is subcutaneous emphysema?

It is a collection of air or gas under the skin, subcutaneous emphysema-crepitus-is usually painless, and feels spongy on palpation. Small amounts of subcutaneous emphysema around the tube insertion site are commonly absorbed. However, if the tube is improperly placed or has an air leak, air may move from the insertion site into the neck, chest, and face and cause pain. The physician needs to be notified if this occurs.[6]

There are several types of chest tubes on the market. The type that is used varies according to individual institutional needs.

Some common types are:

PleuraVac
Heimlich valve
Pleurex catheter

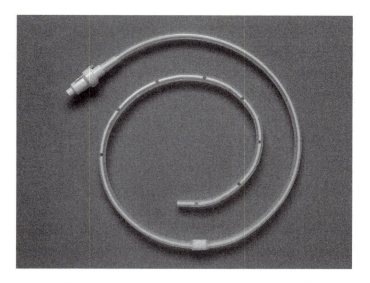

Figure 16.1   **Pleurex catheter.**

All 3 of these devices can be used in the inpatient setting. The Pleurex catheter (**Figure 16.1**) and Heimlich valve can also be used in the home setting. They are easy for the patient to empty and provide for adequate pleural drainage. In addition, these devices allow for the patient to be at home.

MJ's chest tube drainage decreases and the physician orders pleuradisis.

What is pleuradisis?

Pleuradisis is a procedure done to obliterate the pleural space after fluid drainage. A physician performs this procedure by instilling an irritating agent, such as bleomycin or talc, via a chest tube. The chest tube will be clamped for 60 to 120 minutes after instilling the sclerosing agent. The chest tube may be left in for a few days after the sclerosing to promote adherence of the pleura.[6]

For what oncologic emergencies is MJ at risk?

Patients who are diagnosised with lung cancer are at risk for many types of oncology emergencies, such as hypercalcemia, syndrome of inappropriate antidiuretic hormone, spinal cord compression, and superior vena cava syndrome.[7-8]

Describe each of these oncologic emergencies.

Hypercalcemia is a metabolic emergency that occurs as a result of increased bone resorption that may be caused by bone destruction, by tumor invasion, or by increased levels of parathyroid hormone osteoclast activating factor or prostaglandin produced by the tumor.[7]

Syndrome of inappropriate antidiuretic hormone is a metabolic emergency syndrome resulting from the nonphysiologic release of antidiuretic hormone from the posterior pituitary gland or from an exogenous source leading to impaired renal function.[7]

Spinal cord compression is a structural emergency that results in the compression of the spinal cord due to tumor within or on the spinal cord, causing a decreased blood supply and altered neurological function.[8]

Superior vena cava syndrome is a structural emergency that occurs when there is compromise of the venous drainage from the head, neck, upper extremities, and thorax to the heart due to tumor compression or an obstruction of the superior vena cava vessel.[8]

MJ had his chest tube removed 2 days after the pleuradisis. He went home and is starting a new regimen of chemotherapy next week.

A list of lung cancer resources can be found in **Table 16.1**.

REFERENCES

1. Koope CS. Lung cancers. In: Yarbro S, Frogge M, Goodman M, Groenwald SL. *Cancer Principles and Practice.* 6th ed. Sudbury, MA: Jones and Bartlett; 2005:1379-1409.

2. Ginsberg RJ, Volkres EE, Rosenzweig K. Non-small cell lung cancer. In: Devita VT, Hellman S, Rosenberg SA, eds. *Cancer Principles and Practice.* 6th ed. Philadelphia, PA: Lippincott Williams and Wilkins; 2001:925-983.

Table 16.1   **Lung Cancer Resources**

Lung Cancer Alliance
800-298-2436 (Lung Cancer Hotline)
www.alcase.org

American Cancer Society
800-ACS-2345
www.cancer.org

American Lung Association
800-LUNGUSA
www.lungusa.org

American Society of Clinical Oncology
(ASCO)
888-651-3038
www.peoplelivingwithcancer.org

Cancer Care, Inc.
800-813-HOPE
www.cancercare.org

It's Time to Focus on Lung Cancer
877-646-LUNG
www.lungcancer.org

National Cancer Institute
800-4-CANCER
www.nci.nih.gov

Oncology Nursing Society
866-257-4ONS
www.ons.org

The Wellness Community
888-793-WELL
www.thewellnesscommunity.org

OncoLink
Abramson Cancer Center, University of
Pennsylvania
215-349-8895 (Editorial)
www.oncolink.upenn.edu

Quitnet
617-437-1500
www.quitnet.com

3. Greene FL. Lung cancer staging. In: American Cancer Society, American Joint Committee on Cancer. *AJCC Cancer Staging Manual*. 6th ed. New York: Springer-Verlag, Inc; 2002:173-177.

4. Kucharczuk JC, Kaiser LR. Video-assisted thoracic surgery. *Contemporary Surgery*. 2002:58(11):571-574.

5. Flannery M. Lung cancer. In: Itano JK, Taoka KN, eds. *Core Curriculum for Oncology Nursing*. 4th ed. St. Louis, MO: Elsevier Saunders; 2005:512-523.

6. Lazzara D. Eliminate the air of mystery from chest tubes. *Nursing*. 2002;32(6) 36-43.

7. Gobel BH. Metabolic emergencies. In: Itano JK, Taoka KN, eds. *Core Curriculum for Oncology Nursing*. 4th ed. St. Louis, MO: Elsevier Saunders; 2005:383-421.

8. Hunter JC. Structural emergencies. In: Itano JK, Taoka KN, eds. *Core Curriculum for Oncology Nursing*. 4th ed. St. Louis, MO: Elsevier Saunders; 2005:423-439.

17

Safe Chemotherapy Administration Case Study

MW is a 67-year-old female who was diagnosed with non-small cell lung cancer (NSCLC) 15 months ago. She was initially treated with 6 cycles of carboplatin (Paraplatin) and paclitaxel (Taxol) along with 6 weeks of concurrent radiation therapy. She tolerated both of these treatment modalities well and had a marked decrease in her lung cancer related symptoms. MW now presents for additional chemotherapy for a reoccurrence of her disease. She has been experiencing an increase in shortness of breath over the last several months and a CAT scan reveals an increase in the size of her lung tumors compared to one done 3 months ago. Treatment with vinorelbine (Navelbine) and gemcitabine (Gemzar) is scheduled today. MW had a left portacath placed 1 week ago, which is patent, functioning well, and has a brisk blood return. A CBC, SMA 7, BUN and creatinine are ordered prior to the start of chemotherapy. MW never smoked, but her husband of 45 years smokes 2 packs of cigarettes a day and she grew up with a family of smokers. She also tells her nurse that her father and brother died of lung cancer.

What teaching should the nurse do with MW prior to administering her chemotherapy?

It is important for MW to have a good understanding of what side effects to expect and how to manage them. She also needs to know what symptoms to report and have all the necessary contact numbers. This relates strongly to safety because some chemotherapy-related side effects such as neutropenia can be fatal if not appropriately managed. Make sure that she has written information that reinforces any verbal instruction to take home. These concepts apply to any type of chemotherapy regimen. Information about the supportive care services such as social work, nutrition, and support groups should be given at this time if the patient has not already received this information. Many pre-chemotherapy teaching sessions include a tour of the treatment area.

What to teach is based on anticipated side effects. The main side effects of vinorelbine are myelosuppression, particularly neutropenia, mild nausea and vomiting, and mild to moderate neuropathy. The main side effects of gemcitabine include myelosuppression, mild to moderate nausea and vomiting, flu-like symptoms and fever, and edema. Myelosupression, especially neutropenia and thrombocytopenia, is a frequent but short-lived toxicity for both drugs. MW needs to be taught self-care measures to avoid infection and bleeding. Measures to avoid infection include good hand washing, avoiding people with colds or other illnesses, avoiding crowds or crowded places, avoiding anything that could create an opening in the skin such as shaving with a straight razor, and practicing safe food handling. Measures to avoid bleeding include avoiding aspirin or aspirin-containing products, avoiding heavy contact activities or sports, wearing shoes or slippers instead of going barefoot, and shaving with an electric razor. Anemia is less common. Only 20% of patients receiving gemcitabine require a blood transfusion during their course of treatment. Mild to moderate nausea and vomiting can be prevented or controlled with antiemetics. The nurse should teach MW how to take her antiemetics and encourage her to fill her prescription for them before getting nauseous so she can have some on hand. The nurse should make sure MW can afford to fill her prescriptions and refer her to a social worker or other designated person if she cannot. She should encourage small, frequent meals of cool, bland foods and adequate fluid intake. MW should call if she is unable to keep fluids down. Neuropathy from vinorelbine can be in the form of constipation or numbness and tingling in the hands and feet. MW should report either constipation or changes in sensation. If MW already has a history of constipation, a stimulating laxative may be given as a preventative measure. Transient episodes of fever and flulike symptoms occur with 41% of patients receiving gemcitabine. MW should be told that these are possible side effects and she should take acetaminophen (Tylenol) two tablets every four hours as needed to relieve these side effects as directed by her physician. MW should report any swelling if it occurs. Edema occurs in about a third of patients, and it is reversible when the drug is discontinued. Both vinorelbine and gemcitabine cause minimal hair loss. A nurse who is teaching about a drug that caused hair loss should include information for the patient about wigs and hats and the American Cancer Society's Look Good Feel Better Program. This program helps women cope with the physical changes of chemotherapy and teaches them about makeup and wig styling techniques. Hair loss from most chemotherapy drugs can be expected to occur within 21 days. Having this information gives patients time to obtain a wig or hat before the 21 days begins. Females of childbearing age should use contraception since both drugs could cause damage to a fetus.[1]

MW asks if her lung cancer and subsequent reoccurrence are related to the smoking in her household. How should one respond?

Most lung cancer is directly related to cigarette smoking. The risk of developing lung cancer rises with the number of cigarettes smoked a day and number of total years smoked. Each year, approximately 3,000 nonsmoking adults die of lung cancer as a result of second-hand smoke. There is also a combination of other causes that include environmental and genetic factors. MW has a history of exposure to second-hand smoke and we are not able to determine what environmental or genetic factors exist. An appropriate answer would be to say that some lung cancers are due to second-hand smoke but other factors such as the environment and heredity play a role that is unclear at this time.[2]

Prior to giving MW chemotherapy, what would the nurse need to do to assure safety in administration?

An accurate height and weight are necessary to be sure the dose is calculated properly. A height and weight from a previous cycle should not be used because MW may have gained or lost weight since that time. Since the weight is a factor in dosage calculation, a change in weight could result in an incorrect dose unless ideal body weight is being used. The nurse should then check the chemotherapy orders to be sure that they are correct for MW's diagnosis. She should calculate dosages to assure that they are within the accepted dose range, using a reliable source that lists dose ranges approved for each chemotherapy drug. Clinical trial protocol supersedes all other referenced information. Next the nurse should check the lab results to verify that they are within normal limits. She should verify that consent has been signed to be sure that MW has been properly informed of the risks and benefits of her chemotherapy regimen and has been informed of any alternate treatments. Finally, she should verify that MW's port is functioning properly and that she is able to obtain a blood return. Patients who do not have a venous access device need to have a properly functioning IV catheter. Note any premeds or prehydration that needs to be given.[3]

What should one do if MW has not signed a consent form for chemotherapy?

The nurse should inform the physician that consent has not been signed and request that one is completed before she administers the chemotherapy or follows other institutional policies regarding consent.[3]

How does body surface area (BSA) relate to chemotherapy drug calculation?

The BSA is multiplied by the prescribed unit dose per protocol listed as mg/m^2 and will be equal to the dose to be given.[3]

Calculate MW's BSA.

MW's BSA is 1.95.

This number was based on the formula listed in **Figure 17.1** below. Many body surface calculators exist and are reliable, or the calculation can be done using a calculator with square root capability. The use of a nomogram is not recommended because copy machine distortion can exist and affect the dose.[3]

The physician orders are for ondansetron (Zofran) 24 mg IV prechemotherapy, vinorelbine 39 mg (20 mg/m[2]) IV push and gemcitabine 2950 mg (1000 mg/m[2]) over 30 minutes. These drugs are given on days 1 and 8 every 3 weeks for 6 cycles.

What resource could one go to to verify correct dosages for chemotherapy agents?

An up-to-date chemotherapy drug book should contain this information and be readily available in the work area. If the patient is participating in a clinical trial, the schema page of the protocol contains dosage information that is readily available on the chart.[3]

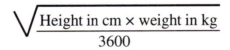

$$\sqrt{\frac{\text{Height in cm} \times \text{weight in kg}}{3600}}$$

Figure 17.1   Calculate BSA.
Source: Polovich M, White JM, Kelleher LO, eds. *2005 Chemotherapy and Biotherapy Guidelines and Recommendations for Practice.* 2nd ed. Pittsburgh, PA: Oncology Nursing Press; 2005:65.

Are these dosages correct? If not, what type of follow-up should the nurse do?

The dose of vinorelbine is correct. Take the patient's BSA of 1.95 and multiply it by 20 mg/m^2 to get the dose of 39 mg. The dose is within the correct dose range for this drug. The dose of gemcitabine is incorrect. Based on MW's BSA, she should receive 1950 mg. Because the dose is higher than the recommended dose for MW, the nurse decides to discuss this with the physician and not go forward with hanging the drug. This also underscores the importance of the double-check procedure for chemotherapy. One should not assume someone else's calculations are correct. There should be a check when the dose is ordered, a check when the dose is mixed, and an independent 2-nurse double check before the chemotherapy is hung.[3]

To reiterate the calculations for MW's dosages:

Vinorelbine 1.95 × 20 = 39 mg
Gemcitabine 1.95 × 1000 = 1950 mg

MW's lab values are as follows: hemoglobin 13 g/dl, hematocrit 38%, WBC 6.2, ANC 2.3, BUN creatinine 1.0 mg/dl.

Are these lab values within normal limits?

Yes, these lab values are within normal limits and it is fine to proceed with the chemotherapy administration process.[1,3]

If the nurse is pregnant, how would that alter her practice?

According to the Occupational Safety and Health Administration (OSHA) guidelines, anyone who is pregnant, actively trying to conceive (men or women), or breast-feeding should not handle chemotherapy agents. This would include mixing and administering chemotherapy agents as well as handling excreta from patients for 48 hours after chemotherapy administration.[3]

The next step is to hang MW's chemotherapy. What final safety measures are still necessary before starting?

The nurse should do an independent double check with another chemotherapy-approved provider that includes BSA, drug, dosage, and lab values to verify that the calculations are accurate. The chemotherapy-approved provider can be an RN, an MD, or a pharmacist as per institutional policy. Most RNs attend an Oncology Nursing Society (ONS)-approved chemotherapy and biotherapy didactic course followed by a skills practicum at their own clinic or institution. The didactic portion and the practicum are both necessary. The nurse should also follow the 5 rights of medication by asking MW her name and date of birth and verifying it against the chemotherapy order. If the patient has an identification bracelet she would use the patient's medical record as an identifier as well.[3] According to the Joint Commission of Accreditation of Healthcare Organizations (JCAHO), the nurse needs to use 2 identifiers when administering medications.[4] After checking that she has the right patient, she checks for the right dose, right route, right time, and the right medication. Once the chemotherapy is checked, the 2 people who verified that the information is correct document according to institutional policy in the patient's medical record.[3]

The nurse then administers the chemotherapy.

Once the chemotherapy has been administered what documentation should be included?

Symptoms experienced during the last chemotherapy treatment and current symptoms the patient is experiencing should be documented. The symptoms are from the patient's perspective and include severity, i.e., mild, moderate, and severe or a number on the 0-10 scale. The nurse should also document the date and time; drug name, dose, and route of administration; volume and type of fluids; assessment of the site before and after infusion; information of the infusion device; verification of blood return before, during, and after therapy; patient and family education; response to treatment; and posttreatment and discharge instructions.[3]

A drop of chemotherapy medicine spills on the nurse's arm as she is administering MW's chemotherapy. What should she do?

She should wash her skin with plain soap and water for at least 5 minutes. If the chemotherapy has gotten on her clothing, she should change clothes, place the contaminated clothing in a plastic bag, take it home and wash it separately from any other laundry. She should let her supervisor know so that proper follow-up can be done and that an incident report can be filled out according to institutional reporting procedures.[3]

What should she do if chemotherapy splashes in her eye?

If chemotherapy medicine splashes into the nurse's eye, she should go to the nearest eye wash station and rinse her eyes with plain water for 15 minutes and then follow procedures for notifying her supervisor. All employees should locate the eye wash station ahead of time.[3]

How can this be prevented from happening in the future?

The nurse should wear a lint-free gown made out of fabric with low permeability to prevent chemotherapy drugs from coming through onto the skin in addition to double gloving with gloves approved for hazardous drugs. Chemotherapy bags can be primed with saline so that spiking the bag does not result in exposure. Finally, policies and procedures regarding chemotherapy safety that nurses are expected to follow should be put into place and reviewed annually.[3]

Are either of MW's chemotherapy agent vesicants?

Yes, vinorelbine is considered a vesicant, so ideally it should be given via a central venous access device. If it is not being given via a central venous access device, the IV should be newly placed and not over an area that contains bones or tendons such as the hand or wrist, or a high movement area such as the antecubital area. All continuous vesicant infusions should be given via a central venous access device. MW has a left portacath. Her nurse would check for catheter patency and assure that she has a brisk blood return prior to administration. She would then administer this drug over no more than 6-10 minutes through the side port of a free-flowing IV closest to the IV bag followed by a flush of 75-125 ml of fluid to reduce the incidence of phlebitis and severe back pain that can occur following vinorelbine administration.[1,3]

What should the nurse do if vinorelbine did extravasate?

She should immediately stop the IVP and saline infusion, disconnect the tubing, and attempt to aspirate any residual drug and blood from the IV tubing and catheter/needle IV site if possible. She should notify the MD. Use of an antidote is controversial and not recommended at this time. She should apply warm soaks. (Most vesicants require cold; nurses should consult a reference book related to each specific agent.) She should elevate the arm and assess the arm for pain, progression of erythema, induration, and evidence of necrosis. She should arrange for follow-up observation and teach MW about signs and symptoms to report. She should take a picture if possible and carefully document the following on the patient's medical record: date, time, insertion site, needle size and type, and drugs administered. The documentation should also include the amount of drug administered prior to the extravasation, interventions, the appearance of the site, and MW's responses. She should include a follow-up plan and give a copy of the plan to MW in writing. The nurse should follow up with reporting the extravasation to her supervisor according to institutional policy.[1,3]

What supplies and equipment should be on hand to assure safe administration of MW's chemotherapy?

The nurse should wear personal protective equipment (PPE) which includes powder-free gloves that have been tested for hazardous drugs; these include latex, nitrile, polyurethane, or neoprene. Double gloving is recommended for all handling activities—the nurse should wear a disposable lint-free gown made of a low permeability fabric with one set of gloves under the gown cuff and one set extending over the gown cuff. Eye and face protection should be used if there is a danger of splashing. A properly labeled, nonpermeable, hazardous-drug container should be stored in an appropriate location for proper disposal of materials used to administer chemotherapy. A chemotherapy spill kit should be readily available. A respirator mask should be used when cleaning spills. Nurses should have access to information about what to do in the event of an exposure; for example, material safety data sheets should be readily available. The institution should have an extravasation kit and emergency equipment available as needed.[3]

REFERENCES

1. Wilkes GM, Barton-Burke M. *2005 Oncology Nursing Drug Handbook*. Sudbury, MA: Jones and Bartlett Publishers; 2005:4, 5, 11, 27-29, 39, 174-178, 310-313.

2. American Cancer Society. *ACS Cancer Facts and Figures—2005*. Atlanta, GA: American Cancer Society; 2005.

3. Polovich M, White JM, Kelleher LO, eds. *2005 Chemotherapy and Biotherapy Guidelines and Recommendations for Practice*. 2nd ed. Pittsburgh, PA: Oncology Nursing Press; 2005:1-13, 53-77, 78-86, 226.

4. Joint Commission on Accreditation of Healthcare Organizations. *Comprehensive accreditation manual for hospitals: the official handbook*. Outlook Terrace, IL: Author; 2004.

18

Sexuality Case Study

MS is a 32-year-old female diagnosed with stage III breast cancer. She is status post-right lumpectomy with axillary node dissection, which was done following a positive sentinel node biopsy. A chemotherapy nurse is teaching MS about what to expect with her planned chemotherapy treatment in a pre-chemotherapy teaching class. Her husband is present and appears very supportive. The nurse learns that they have been married for 6 months and have no children. MS will be receiving 4 cycles of dose-dense doxorubicin (Adriamycin) and cyclophosphamide (Cytoxan) followed by 4 cycles of paclitaxel (Taxol). The nurse discusses side effects with MS, such as risk for developing neutropenia, fatigue, nausea and vomiting, hair loss, myalgia, and neuropathy. MS is very concerned about being able to get pregnant once treatment is completed. She says that she is concerned about her survival. She confides that both issues are weighing heavily on her. When her husband leaves the room she also confides that she is concerned that her surgical scars and loss of hair will be unattractive to her husband. She says that she cannot look at her surgical scars.

How should MS's concerns be addressed?

There are actually several issues that the nurse needs to begin to address with MS, including fertility, body image, and survival. They are all interrelated. The most immediate issue that her nurse needs to address is fertility. Chemotherapy could, in fact, affect MS's fertility either on a temporary or permanent basis. Part of informed consent consists of making sure that MS is aware of that and that she is aware of what her options are. Age is a factor, as are type of treatment, dose of treatment, and length of time posttreatment. Single-agent chemotherapy is less toxic to the ovaries than combination therapy. The ovaries of women younger than 35 can tolerate greater doses of chemotherapy. Alkylating agents are thought to be the most damaging to fertility because they can cause ovarian failure.[1] Alkylating agents include altretamine (Hexalen), busulfan (Myleran), carboplatin (Paraplatin), chlorambucil (Leukeran), cisplatin (Platinol), cyclophosphamide, dacarbazine (DTIC), ifosfamide (Ifex), mechlorethamine (nitrogen mustard, Mustargen), melphalan (Alkeran), oxaliplatin (Eloxatin), temozolomide (Temodar), and thiotepa (Thioplex).[2] For additional information on chemotherapeutic agents affecting sexual or reproductive function, see **Table 18.1**.

The nurse refers MS to a reproductive gynecologist to discuss potential options. Some options include in vitro fertilization, gamete intrafallopian transfer, use of donor oocytes, having a surrogate gestational carrier or surrogate mother, cryopreservation and embryo banking, embryo donation, adoption, and child-free living.[2] Many factors comprise sexuality. As many as 40%-100% of patients report some evidence of sexual dysfunction following chemotherapy. This symptom is underreported because doctors and nurses do not routinely assess it and patients do not always feel comfortable addressing it first.[3]

The next issue is survival. This is a very common concern for patients at diagnosis, throughout treatment, and following treatment. Many cancer centers have programs and support groups for cancer survivors in which MS could participate. In addition, there are online resources that could be of benefit to MS, such as the National Coalition for Cancer Survivorship, found at www.canceradvocacy.org.

Table 18.1   Chemotheraputic Agents Affecting Sexual or Reproductive Function

Agent	Complications
Alkylating Agents	
Altretamine Busulfan Chlorambucil Cisplatin Cyclophosphamide Ifosfamide Melphalan Nitrogen mustard	Amenorrhea, oligospermia, azoospermia, decreased libido, ovarian dysfunction, erectile dysfunction
Antimetabolites	
Cytosine arabinoside Fludarabine phosphate 5-Fluorouracil Methotrexate	As for alkylating agents
Antitumor Antibiotics	
Dactinomycin Daunorubicin Doxorubicin Plicamycin	As for alkylating agents
Plant Products	
Vinblastine Vincristine	Decreased libido, ovarian dysfunction, erectile dysfunction Retrograde ejaculation, erectile dysfunction
Miscellaneous Agents	
Aminoglutethimide Androgens Antiandrogens Antiestrogens Corticosteroids Estrogens Goserelin acetate Interferons Procarbazine Progestins	Irregular menses, acne Masculinization (women) Decreased libido, impotence Gynecomastia, impotence Transient impotence Gynecomastia, acne Impotence Amenorrhea, pelvic pain As for alkylating agents Menstrual abnormalities, change in libido, masculinization (women)

Source: Krebs LU. Sexual and reproductive dysfunction. In: Yarbro CH, Frogge MH, Goodman M, eds. *Cancer Nursing Principles and Practice.* 6th ed. Sudbury, MA: Jones and Bartlett; 2006:854.

The final issue is an issue about body image. MS has concerns about the changes in her appearance and how it will affect her attractiveness to her husband. There are many supportive options for MS that will help her address these 3 issues. It is important that the nurse be present and be willing to listen to her concerns. A non-threatening environment is essential. The nurse should provide MS with information about support groups that could help her deal with issues of sexuality and body image. A young women's cancer support group is one example. Many women benefit from individual or group counseling with a psychologist. Other women benefit from support groups with a dietician and physical therapist that focus on diet and exercise. Still others will benefit from integrative therapies such as music therapy, Shiatsu massage, and art therapy.

Three months after chemotherapy is completed, MJ is complaining of severe hot flashes and depression. What might be occurring?

MS is experiencing signs and symptoms of chemotherapy-induced menopause because of the ovarian suppression related to chemotherapy. There is a diminished amount of estrogen in MS's body. This has a direct effect on the hypothalamus, the part of the brain responsible for controlling appetite, sleep cycles, sex hormones, and body temperature.

Symptoms of estrogen loss include decreased libido, hot flashes, sleep disruption, mood changes including anxiety and depression, trouble making decisions, vaginal changes, dryness, itching, burning, painful intercourse, vaginal or bladder infections, headache, dizziness, skin changes, and thinning of scalp and pubic hair. Only 10%-15% of women experience severe hot flashes. Most are mild to moderate. The drop in estrogen confuses the hypothalamus and makes it read "too hot." The brain then responds by sending an instant alert to the heart, blood vessels, and nervous system to get the heat out. The heart pumps faster, the blood vessels in the skin dilate to circulate more blood to radiate off the heat, and sweat glands release more sweat. Hot flashes can last from a few seconds to up to an hour. They begin as menopause approaches and can continue for many more years after periods stop. If a patient is taking an anti-estrogen agent such as tamoxifen (Nolvadex) or an aromatase inhibitor such as anastrozole (Arimidex), letrozole (Femara), or exemestane (Aromasin) the intensity of hot flashes improves after the first 3-6 months. Thin women or women who smoke may experience more severe hot flashes.[1,3] **Table 18.2** provides guidelines for dealing with hot flashes.

What are some other treatment-related causes of menopause?

Other causes include surgical removal of the ovaries, hormone-blocking agents, and radiation.[1]

What should the nurse teach MS about hot flashes?

The nurse should instruct MS to avoid hot flash triggers. One way for women to learn what their triggers are is to keep a hot flash log. In general, things to avoid include stress, spicy foods, alcohol, caffeine, hot foods, refined sugar, smoking, tight clothing, hot weather, saunas, hot tubs, and hot showers.

Table 18.2   **Hot Flash Survival Tips**

- Take vitamin E 200-800 IU a day.
- Dress in layers.
- Wear loosely woven cotton or rayon clothes including at night.
- Use cotton sheets.
- Lower the thermostat, use AC, a ceiling fan, or handheld fan.
- Try relaxation exercises, deep breathing, guided imagery, hypnosis, biofeedback, and acupuncture. These integrative modalities have been helpful to some women.

Source: Polovich M, White JM, Kelleher LO, eds. *2005 Chemotherapy and Biotherapy Guidelines and Recommendations for Practice.* 2nd ed. Pittsburgh, PA: Oncology Nursing Press; 2005:203.

MS asks if she can take an herbal remedy or soy supplements to help manage the effects of her hot flashes. How can the nurse respond?

Many herbal remedies contain plant estrogen and are not recommended. Some herbal remedies include soy, evening primrose, black cohosh, angelica, ginseng, and licorice root. Dietary soy is fine but soy or flax supplements are not recommended. Estrogen replacement is not usually indicated for women who are experiencing menopause because of interventions to prevent breast cancer or those who have hormone-responsive cancers. Some low-dose estrogen vaginal crèmes are appropriate. Instruct MS not to begin any new medications, including over-the-counter ones, without consulting with her doctor first.[3]

What is used for the medical management of severe hot flashes?

Blood pressure lowering medications such as clonidine (Catapres-TTS) lessen the frequency and severity of hot flashes by modifying the blood vessels' response to the brain's signal to give off heat. Antidepressants in low doses may stop a hot flash by rebalancing or intercepting epinephrine and serotonin—the brain chemicals that transmit the hot flash alarm.[3]

The websites in **Table 18.3** can help women who are of childbearing age and receiving chemotherapy deal with issues such as fertility and chemotherapy induced menopause.

Table 18.3   **Sexuality Web Sites**

Fertile Hope—fertility resources for cancer patients
www.fertilehope.org

North American Menopause Society
www.menopause.org

Power Surge: A Warm and Caring Community for Women in Menopause
www.power-surge.com

REFERENCES

1. Lynch MP. *Essentials of Oncology Care*. New York: Professional Publishing Group; 2005:150-153.

2. Polovich M, White JM, Kelleher LO, eds. *2005 Chemotherapy and Biotherapy Guidelines and Recommendations for Practice*. 2nd ed. Pittsburgh, PA: Oncology Nursing Press; 2005:20-22.

3. Polovich M, White JM, Kelleher LO, eds. *2005 Chemotherapy and Biotherapy Guidelines and Recommendations for Practice*. 2nd ed. Pittsburgh, PA: Oncology Nursing Press; 2005:198-205.

19

Spinal Cord Compression Case Study

MJ is an 80-year-old male who presents in the ER. His chief complaints are lower back pain, weakness, and difficulty ambulating. He is also complaining of back pain for the last 2 weeks that is unrelieved by oxycodone and acetaminophen (Percocet). He is accompanied by his wife, who states that he has fallen 3 times in the past few days. He is complaining of right knee pain. His knee is swollen and bruised. MJ has a history of prostate cancer that was diagnosed 15 years ago. He has been symptom free until 2 weeks ago when he was golfing and he felt some back discomfort that has gotten worse. The weakness in his legs and his difficulty in ambulating has progressively gotten worse over the past 4 days. MJ and his wife have 4 children who live close to their parents.

What assessments should the nurse do?

The nurse should obtain a history from MJ, knowing that his particular type of cancer and his symptoms may make him considered high risk for an oncology emergency. He would need to have his pain assessed, focusing on location, intensity, and other factors such as radiating pain. Neck and back pain are often one of the first signs of spinal cord compression. Pain is usually worse in the supine position and aggravated by movement. MJ needs a neurological assessment since he is complaining of trouble ambulating and has had recent falls. The nurse should check for loss of sensation for deep pressure, position, and vibrations.

The nurse examines MJ's right knee and assesses his range of motion (ROM) and skin integrity. He assesses MJ's functional status and home situation related to safety and in preparation for discharge planning in the future.[1] He assesses MJ's bowel and bladder function to see if he has symptoms of incontinence. He states he has had some dribbling and frequency with urination. He tells his nurse he has had some urinary incontinence.

He denies incontinence of his bowels at this time.

The nurse assesses for paralysis, sexual impotence, and muscle atrophy.

He also asks MJ about his falls and the participating factors surrounding his falls. MJ says his legs just gave out from under him.

The nurse asks MJ about his oxycodone and acetaminophen usage over the past 2 weeks.[1]

What oncologic emergency might MJ be experiencing? What suggests this emergency?

MJ has all the classic signs and symptoms of a spinal cord compression (SCC). He has a history of prostate cancer, back pain, an unsteady gait with recent falls and he is complaining of some urinary incontinence.[1-2]

The physician examines MJ and he orders the following diagnostic tests:

Spinal X-rays
CT scan of the spine
MRI of the spine
X-ray of the right knee

What preprocedural teaching should the nurse do with MJ?

The nurse explains to MJ the reasons for his upcoming tests. The X-ray of his right knee is to check for a fracture since he had a recent fall. The spinal X-rays are to check for fractures and soft tissue damage. The MRI is ordered to assist in the diagnosis of SCC and evaluating the degree of cord compression. The CAT scan will examine vertebral stability and bone loss and destruction.[1-2]

None of these tests require any specific preparation but it might be best to ask MJ if he is claustrophobic since the MRI and CAT scan can make a patient feel claustrophobic. If MJ is claustrophobic, then he might require sedation prior to the MRI to decrease his anxiety. The MRI will also be a noisy procedure and he will wear earplugs and hear a banging noise.

What additional action should the nurse consider prior to sending MJ off to radiology?

The nurse should medicate MJ for pain since movement is painful for him and these tests require movement getting on and off the radiology tables.

MJ goes for his tests and the CAT scan and MRI show that he has SCC. The X-ray of his right knee is negative.

What is spinal cord compression?

SCC is a compression of the spinal cord and is considered an oncology emergency. It occurs when tumors within the spinal cord or vertebral column metastasize, causing pressure and compression on the tissue and blood supply of the spinal cord resulting in neurological symptoms. Patients will exhibit signs and symptoms similar to those experienced by MJ. The initial symptoms are usually mild, but must be recognized early by clinicians, because if they are not promptly treated, SCC can result in permanent neurological deficits for the patient.[1]

It is important to be aware of locations of metastasis to the spine, especially in patients who have a cancer that is likely to metastasize to the spine who have complaints of back pain.

The treatment most often used for treatment of spinal cord compression is which of the following?

A. Steroids
B. Radiation therapy

C. Pain medication

D. Nutrition therapy

Radiation therapy is the treatment of choice for SCC. Although other therapies may be used, radiation therapy is the most common treatment for cord compression and epidural metastasis if the tumor is known to be radiosensitive and the spine is stable. The other treatments listed may also be used as treatment in conjunction with the radiation therapy.[1]

MJ is admitted to the nursing unit for prompt treatment of his SCC. He is started on a morphine patient-controlled analgesia (PCA) pump at 0.5 mg/hour basal rate with 1 mg q 20 minutes for breakthrough pain.

Which 3 nursing diagnoses are priorities for MJ?

Alteration in comfort—MJ has acute pain in his back for the past 2 weeks unrelieved by oral medications and is on a morphine PCA. Since MJ is on a narcotic, he should also be placed on a bowel program to prevent constipation.

Impaired mobility—MJ has difficulty ambulating and has weakness in his lower extremities. He has a recent history of falls.

Impaired urinary elimination—MJ is complaining of dribbling and frequency with some incontinence.

What should the nurse include in his plan of care for MJ?

Pain management is a priority since he wants to get MJ comfortable. Patient safety is another priority based on MJ's presenting symptoms and history. MJ and his family should receive education related to the plan of care including medications, treatments, and discharge planning.

The radiation oncologist sees MJ. He recommends radiation therapy over several weeks at a dose of 3000 cGY, as it is the treatment of choice for SCC.[2] He orders PCA morphine for MJ's pain. He rates his back pain as 7 on a 0-10 scale. MJ states he is not getting much pain relief. As mentioned previously, he is receiving a basal dose of morphine of 0.5 mg/hr and a PCA dose of morphine of 1 mg q 20 minutes for breakthrough pain. His physician increases the basal rate to 1 mg/hr. He starts dexamethasone (Decadron) 100 mg IV q 6 hours. MJ will begin physical therapy.

What should the nurse teach MJ and his wife about his radiation treatment?

The nurse explains to MJ and his wife that radiation therapy is a local treatment to help alleviate his symptoms and decrease his pain. He explains what will happen to MJ during his radiation treatments, including the simulation process and ongoing treatments. They should plan for the simulation session to take at least 1 hour. MJ will receive patient education material related to radiation therapy at the hospital. MJ will receive 20 treatments over a 4-week period.

Which side effects should the nurse assess for?

MJ's nurse should assess MJ for fatigue, bone marrow depression, skin changes in the radiation field, and changes in bowel or bladder function.[1-2]

What should the nurse teach MJ and his wife about his medications?

MJ's nurse reviews the purpose and side effects of dexamethasone and morphine. The dexamethasone is used to reduce inflammation and edema, as well as pain. He teaches MJ the importance of taking his medications as ordered and not to abruptly stop dexamethasone since it is a medication that needs to be tapered before stopping. The morphine is for MJ's back pain.

What other medications should be ordered?

MJ should be on a bowel program since a major side effect of opioid use is constipation. He will need to take a stool softener and a stimulating laxative daily.[3]

MJ becomes confused one night. He does not know where he is and tries to climb out of bed (OOB). He has received 3 doses of dexamethasone prior to this event.

To what can this sudden change in MJ's condition be attributed?

The sudden confusion experienced by MJ is due to the steroids. Some patients receiving steroids develop a steroid-induced psychosis. MJ received a high dose of dexamethasone. The nurse should question the dosage because the usual dosage of dexamethasone is between 4 and 10 mg IV q 6 hours. MJ is also an older adult and is out of his normal environment. MJ is also receiving morphine, which might also be a contributing factor in his change of mental status.[1,3]

What nursing interventions can the nurse implement?

The nurse consults the physician to see if his medications could be the cause of MJ's change in mental status. He assures MJ's safety by making sure he is close to the nurses' station and can be observed frequently. His call bell needs to be within reach and he will need frequent reorientation. If necessary, someone from MJ's family or a sitter should stay with him until this passes. All of his side rails need to be up to help prevent MJ from falling. The nurse could use a bed alarm to alert him when MJ is trying to get OOB. The nurse wants to refrain from using any type of sedation until he knows the cause of MJ's confusion. MJ should be placed on fall precautions since he is at risk for falls.

MJ recovers and his pain is better but he will need to go home on oral pain medications. His physician wants to convert him to oral morphine for discharge. In a 24-hour period, MJ used 48 mg of IV morphine.

On how much oral morphine should MJ be discharged? (Note: 3 mg of oral morphine is roughly equivalent to 1 mg of IV morphine)

Since MJ used 48 mg of IV morphine in a 24-hour period, the method of calculation is to multiply 48 by 3, which is 144 mg of oral morphine in a 24-hour period. The nurse could select sustained-release morphine such as MS Contin every 8 hours. That means he divides the total daily dose by 3 to get 48 mg sustained-release morphine every 8 hours. Sustained-release morphine comes in 30 mg and 15 mg tablets. MJ will take 45 mg oral sustained-release morphine every 8 hours. A breakthrough pain medication is still necessary for episodic pain.

Table 19.1   Pain Reference Card

Initial Pain Assessment

Believe the patient's report of pain

Location: Identify and assess all pain sites

Words to describe pain: Possible neuropathic pain: Sharp, stabbing, shooting, burning. Possible somatic/visceral pain: Throbbing, dull, aching, crampy

Duration: Constant or intermittent? When did it start? Good days and bad days?

Aggravating or alleviating factors: Pain with movement? Pain at rest? Pain unprovoked?

Pain intensity:

	Mild	Moderate	Severe

No pain   0   1   2   3   4   5   6   7   8   9   10   *Worst imaginable*

Pain Treatment

Analgesia selection:

	NSAIDs	Adjuvants	Opioids
Pain rated 1-4: **Mild pain:**	➡	➡	sometimes
Pain rated 5-6: **Moderate pain:**	➡	➡	usually
Pain rated 7-10: **Severe pain:**	sometimes	➡	always

Notes:

❖ **When changing opioids or route, use the equianalgesic table to calculate the dose.**
  Oral morphine dose is **3 times the IV dose.**
  Oral hydromorphone dose is **5 times the IV dose.**
  IV hydromorphone is 1/6th the IV morphine dose.

❖ Because of incomplete cross-tolerance:
  Begin the new opioid drug at 2/3 of the calculated equianalgesic dose.

❖ Rescue doses are immediate-release preparations given at appropriate intervals for pain not controlled by maintenance dose. **Rescue dose is 10% of the daily dose.**

❖ Lower doses are suggested for **geriatric** patients.

❖ Adjunctive medications may benefit certain pain syndromes (tricyclic antidepressants and/or anticonvulsants for neuropathic pain or NSAIDs for inflammatory pain).

❖ Always prescribe a bowel regimen with opioid administration.

❖ Contact the pharmacy with dosing questions.

Source: University of Pennsylvania Health System Continuous Quality Improvement Department.

Table 19.1   **Pain Reference Card (*continued*)**

Opioid Equianalgesic Doses*

Drug	po/pr (mg)	sq/IV (mg)
Morphine immediate release	30	10
Morphine sustained release	30	na
Hydromorphone	7.5	1.5
Oxycodone sustained release	20	na
Oxycodone immediate release	20	na
Codeine	200	130
not recommended Meperidine	300	75

Example: Convert 320 mg/day of IV morphine to IV hydromorphone
From the Opioid Equianalgesic Doses table, note the ratio between hydromorphone and
morphine is 1.5:10

X mg/day of hydromorphone is to 320 mg/day of morphine **as**:
1.5 mg of hydromorphone is to 10 mg of morphine

> $$\frac{X \text{ mg/day hydromorphone}}{320 \text{ mg/day morphine}} = \frac{1.5 \text{ mg hydromorphone}}{10 \text{ mg morphine}}$$
>
> *Cross-multiply:* $10 \times X = 1.5$ times $320 = $ **480**
> *Divide* $480 \div 10 = X = $ **48**
> *Multiply by 2/3:* **48** $\times 2/3 = $ **32** mg/day hydromorphone
> *Divide by 24 to convert daily to hourly*

Fentanyl Patch to Morphine†

Fentanyl mcg/hr transdermal	Morphine mg/24 hrs po (range)	Morphine mg/24 hrs IM/IV (range)
25	45 (30-75)	15 (10-25)
50	90 (76-117)	30 (26-39)
75	135 (118-150)	45 (39-50)
100	180 (151-195)	60 (51-65)
125	225 (196-240)	75 (66-80)
150	270 (241-285)	90 (81-95)
40 mcg/hr fentanyl = 1 mg/hr IV morphine		

Fentanyl patch is *not* recommended for opioid-naive patients.
Fentanyl patch has a delay in onset of action 14-24 hr once applied
Fentanyl patch has a residual effect for 14-24 hrs once removed
Fentanyl patch delivers at an hourly rate and can be considered continuous sq infusion

---

*Agency for Health Care Policy and Research (AHCPR) *Management of Cancer Pain. Clinical Practice Guideline, No 9, AHCPR Pub No. 94-0592,* Rockville, MD; March 1994, U.S. Department of Health and Human Services, Public Health Service.

†Donner B. Zenz M, Tryba M et al. Direct conversion from oral morphine to transdermal fentanyl: a multicenter study in patients with cancer pain. *Pain.* 1996;64:527-534.

Source: University of Pennsylvania Health System Continuous Quality Improvement Department.

The breakthrough dose is roughly a tenth of the total daily dose given every 4 hours as needed. One tenth of 144 mg is 14.4 mg. Immediate release morphine (MSIR) 15 mg can be given as a breakthrough medication.[3] **Table 19.1** can help nurses accurately assess and treat pain.

What discharge planning should be done for MJ?

MJ and his wife should have a social worker consultation to assess their needs for home care. The nurse will need to know MJ's functional status and home situation to assess whether he can go home with home care and physical therapy (PT) or if he would need to go to a nursing facility such as a rehabilitation or skilled nursing unit for further treatment. MJ should also be put on a bowel regimen with a stool softener and a stimulating laxative since he is going home on narcotics. The nurse needs to assess the ability of getting MJ back and forth to complete his radiation treatments.

REFERENCES

1. Hunter JC. Structural emergencies. In: Itano JK, Taoka KN, eds. *Core Curriculum for Oncology Nursing.* 4th ed. St. Louis, MO: Elsevier Saunders; 2005: 426-430.

2. Wilkes GM. Neurological disturbances. In: Yarbro CH, Frogge MH, Goodman M, eds. *Cancer Symptom Management.* 2nd ed. Sudbury, MA: Jones and Bartlett; 1999:344-381.

3. Pasero C, Portenoy RK, McCaffery M. Opioid analgesics. In: McCaffrey M, Pasero C. *Pain: Clinical Manual.* 2nd ed. St. Louis, MO: Mosby; 1999:161-299.

20

Spirituality Case Study

JS is a 75-year-old male who has been recently diagnosed with advanced stage prostate cancer. He is being treated with hormonal therapy and radiation. He is a poor surgical candidate due to a previous cardiac history and the extent of his disease. JS is beginning his third week of radiation and had competed 3 months of hormonal treatments before starting his radiation treatment. JS's side effects include weight gain from the hormonal treatment and incontinence and impotence from radiation. A nurse in the radiation therapy department has developed a positive rapport with JS. Today he told the nurse that he has started going to church for the first time in 20 years. He related to the nurse that "This cancer has been difficult to accept and the side effects are terrible." He says that he has gained some comfort from attending church again and finds that the cancer experience has allowed him to appreciate things that he had been taking for granted prior to his diagnosis.

What might JS be experiencing? Please explain.

JS may be experiencing spiritual distress. Patients frequently examine their spiritual natures when confronted with life-threatening illness. This can be expressed as a relationship with God or higher power but it can also be about nature, art, music, family, or community. These are the beliefs and values that give a person a sense of meaning and purpose in life.[1] Victor Frankel, a psychologist and con-centration camp survivor, describes spirituality as the part in humans that is always free to choose and that can find meaning regardless of the external situa-tion.[2] Tapping into the will to find meaning in difficult situations can help people endure them and may actually help them have the potential to grow. So from a spiritual perspective, patients with cancer struggle to find the inner resources to cope with their experiences with discomfort, suffering, and sometimes even death.

Why is it important for nurses to address spiritual issues?

According to Albaugh, one's spiritual nature is an important component in finding meaning in an experience that contains suffering.[3] Addressing spirituality is another aspect of the caring that defines nursing. While it is important for nurses to be familiar with the practices associated with the major religions, it is even more important to remember that spirituality is as individual as each human being is. Frequently, cancer patients struggle to find meaning in their diagnosis. It is important for nurses to address spiritual issues when treating the whole patient. The mind, the body, and the spirit are interconnected. Therefore, spirituality is an important component of a patient's physical and mental health.

What should the nurse include in a spiritual assessment?

The first step is to ask JS what his faith is or his beliefs are. Next, she needs to assess how important that faith or those beliefs are to him. She should then ask if he is part of a religious or spiritual community. Finally, she should ask if JS would like her to address any issues at this time. She should remember that spiritual assessment is ongoing and is not just done once.[1]

How can nurses facilitate and enhance patients' spiritual journeys?

Nurses can facilitate and enhance patients' spiritual journeys by supporting and accommodating individual needs and by giving patients permission to discuss their concerns. Being present is as important as "doing for" patients with spiritual needs. Nurses can also involve an interdisciplinary team as needed. It is also important for nurses to be aware of what specific resources are available to patients where they work and in the community, such as a chaplain or social worker, as well as their contact information.[4]

What are some barriers to open communication between nurses and patients regarding spirituality?

Some barriers to discussing spirituality with patients include nurses or other health care providers who have not explored their own belief systems and are exhibiting bias when interacting with patients, lack of knowledge or discomfort of the nurse or other health care team member in discussing spiritual issues, and climates that are unsupportive of a patient's individual spiritual needs.[3]

What are some indications that a patient may be in spiritual distress?

A patient who is socially withdrawn or isolated might be experiencing such distress. Such patients might also express anger directed at God, other people, or themselves. They might also exhibit expressions of fear, depression, grief, hopelessness, or despair. Some patients grieve for loss of what once was or experience anxiety and fear related to diagnosis, treatment, pain, the future, the unknown, dying, and the future of loved ones. They might have feelings of guilt, anger, or sorrow about past actions, decisions, life choices, or relationships.[4]

How might the nurse handle a situation where her religious beliefs strongly conflicted with a patient's beliefs?

The nurse should be in touch with her own spiritual beliefs and how those beliefs impact the kind of care that she gives. She should respect a patient's privacy regarding spiritual beliefs. She must not impose her beliefs on others.[1]

REFERENCES

1. Puchalski C, Romer AL. Taking a spiritual history allows clinicians to understand patients more fully. *J Palliat Med.* 2000;3:(1):129-137.

2. Frankel V. *Man's Search for Meaning.* New York: Washington Square Press; 1968.

3. Deshotels J. Spirituality. In: Kuebler KK, Esper P, eds. *Palliative Practices from A-Z for the Bedside Clinician.* Pittsburgh, PA: Oncology Nursing Press; 2002:227-230.

4. Albaugh JA. Spirituality and life threatening illness: a phenomenologic study. *Oncol Nurs Forum.* 2003;30(4):590-598.

21

Stem Cell Transplant Case Study

MG is a 60-year-old female diagnosed with multiple myeloma. She was treated with VAD (vincristine [Oncovin], doxorubicin [Adriamycin], and dexamethasone [Decadron]) for 6 cycles and is now ready for autologous peripheral blood stem cell transplant (APBSCT). MG and her family come to the center from out of state for a multidisciplinary intake session. She has many questions regarding the APBSCT process. MG is a Jehovah's Witness and is at this center because of its bloodless medicine and surgery program.

What does treating a patient in the bloodless medicine and surgery service involve?

Bloodless medicine and surgery involves treating patients without transfusion support. A patient may refuse blood transfusions based on religious, cultural, and/or personal reasons. Patients are supported with medications and techniques during their hospitalization to limit blood loss. Invasive procedures are limited or structured to conserve blood. In addition, prior to any procedure, a patient's blood cell counts are built up as much as possible so that any blood loss will have a minimal effect on the patient.[1]

What can the nurse explain to MG and her family regarding the APBSCT process? MG is of Spanish descent and speaks limited English.

Since MG speaks limited English, a trained medical interpreter will be present at the initial intake session. The nurse should encourage as many family members as possible to attend the intake session so that they also hear the same message. MG is provided with appropriate educational material in Spanish to reinforce the teaching.[2]

The nurse explains what happens in the various phases of the APBSCT. The first step after MG is cleared for transplant is mobilization. During this phase, the patient is given injections of growth factors such as filgrastim (Neupogen) to stimulate the bone marrow to produce large amounts of stem cells. The growth factor encourages stem cells' growth, therefore making them more prevalent in the peripheral circulation. The stem cell collection process involves circulation of blood through an apheresis machine via a triple lumen central catheter. The rest of the blood is circulated back into the body. This procedure takes 4-8 hours daily for 1-4 days until enough stem cells are collected. The actual amount of cells needed depends upon the patient's height and weight. After the collection, the stem cells are stored frozen until they are needed for infusion at a later date.[3] The second step involves the administration of high-dose chemotherapy followed by the infusion of the stem cells back in to the body. The chemotherapy will be given on the first day, and, since MG has multiple myeloma, the stem cell reinfusion will take place on the third day. Usually within 2 weeks, the cells find their way back into the bone marrow and they start to mature and are released into the body as red blood cells, white blood cells, and platelets. During this time period is when MG will feel the most fatigued because her blood counts will be extremely low and because this is when she is most prone to infection and other side effects of treatment such as mouth sores and decreased appetite. Patients usually start to feel better in about 2 weeks. The red blood cells come back first, followed by the white blood cells, and then the platelets. Full recovery usually occurs in about 3 months.[4]

The nurse clearly emphasizes that MG's wishes regarding blood transfusions will be respected at all times. She will be supported with medications to prevent bleeding and growth factors to stimulate blood cell production throughout the transplant process. Invasive or nonessential procedures will be limited. Blood will be drawn using pediatric tubes. Other strategies to minimize blood loss such as less frequent blood drawing will be utilized.

MG has completed her stem cell mobilization and collection and she is admitted to the oncology unit for an APBSCT. The nursing admission history shows that MG has a husband and 2 grown children. She is from out of state and her family will not be staying with MG during her APBSCT as they need to continue working. They will visit on the weekends.

Because MG speaks limited English, what communication methods will the English-speaking nurse use?

The nurse needs to continue to use a trained medical interpreter. Most hospitals have a list of interpreters. The nurse could supplement communication language cards that are commercially available or hand made with the help of her family.[2] There are also phones available for communications that will interpret for the medical staff and the patient.[5]

The nurse has never had experience caring for a Jehovah's Witness patient. How can she learn more about the care for this type of patient?

It is important that she is culturally sensitive and respects this patient's wishes. She asks the patient to explain his/her beliefs to her, especially regarding blood and blood transfusions. She could read more about this religion. Most hospital librarians could help do a literature search. She could ask her clinical educator or pastoral care department to provide her with additional information. Since she knows about this patient's admission prior to hospitalization, she could research this ahead of time so that she is adequately prepared to care for this type of patient. She must include this information in the patient's plan of care. According to Jehovah's Witness philosophy, "Taking blood into body through mouth or veins violates God's laws." However, Jehovah's Witnesses do not consider stem cells blood as they are immature blood cells, and they will accept them

Table 21.1   **Nonblood Management Techniques**

Patients may choose a nonblood approach to care prior to elective (nonemergency) surgery or as a result of traumatic injuries. The medical team will recommend or use certain techniques and technologies including:

- Diet management
- Medications
- Anesthesia techniques
- Surgical methods to minimize blood loss and conserve blood

Diet Management

Diet and nutrition are extremely important for patients considering a nonblood treatment plan. For example, patients may receive recommendations prior to surgery to:

- maintain a nutritious diet high in iron to increase the amount of iron in their blood.
- take other iron supplements such as ferrous sulfate or ferrous gluconate.
- increase intake of vitamin C so the iron is absorbed more effectively.
- take other vitamin supplements such as B_{12} or folic acid.

Medications

The body may require certain medications to help increase red or white blood cells or hemoglobin levels. Medications may also assist with minimizing blood loss and maximizing the amount of oxygen in the blood.

Some medications that may be administered are:

- Oxygen carriers, including perfluorocarbons and hemoglobin substitutes
- Aprotinin
- Aminocaproic acid
- Desmopressin
- Vasopressin
- Vitamin K

In addition, the physician may request that patients stop taking other medications, such as aspirin or anti-inflammatory drugs. Some medications may hinder blood counts or clotting abilities. If the patient is a smoker, he or she will be strongly urged to stop smoking because it can interfere with oxygen delivery throughout the body.

Anesthesia Techniques

The medical team may use certain anesthesia techniques during surgery, including:

- Volume expanders (crystalloids/colloids)
- Hypotensive anesthesia
- Hypothermia
- Normovolemic hemodilution

Table 21.1   **Nonblood Management Techniques** (*continued*)

Surgical Methods
Surgical methods to minimize blood loss or conserve blood may include using pediatric tubes, limiting blood sampling, or using pharmaceuticals. The staff uses a variety of surgical devices to limit blood loss, including:

- Electrocautery
- Ultrasonic scalpel
- Laser surgery
- Argon beam coagulator
- Autotransfusion devices
- Selective embolization

Source: The Center for Bloodless Medicine and Surgery at Pennsylvania Hospital. Non-blood management techniques. Available at: http://pennhealth.com/bloodless/management.htm#diet. Accessed August 1, 2006.

for transplant.[1] Techniques for nonblood management can be found in **Table 21.1**.

MG is 5 feet 6 inches feet tall and weighs 160 lbs. She is allergic to penicillin. Her physical exam is unremarkable at this time. Her vital signs are stable. MG is admitted and will be treated with melphalan (Alkeran) on the day of admission.

Admission orders include the following:

Daily weights and abdominal girth
Notify MD for a 2-lb or greater weight gain
Daily CBC with differential, SMA-10 and LFTs, magnesium level at 6 am
    daily unless otherwise noted
Daily urinalysis
Use pediatric blood tubes for all blood draws
Daily EKG
Neutropenic precautions
Peridex mouth care 5 times daily
Consult social work, physical therapy and nutrition

VS q 4 hours. Notify MD for temperature greater than 100.5°F

Strict recording of intake and output. Notify MD if intake/output are unequal.

Urine pH after each void

Incentive spirometry q 4 hours while awake

Ondansetron (Zofran) 24 mg pre-chemotherapy

Dexamethasone 20 mg IV

Lorazepam (Ativan) 1 mg pre-chemotherapy and q 6 hours prn for nausea and vomiting

Notify MD for any nausea and vomiting

Oxycodone and acetaminophen (Percocet) 2 tablets po q 4 hours prn pain

Fluconazole (Diflucan) 100 mg orally daily starting on day of reinfusion

Histamine H2 antagonist daily starting on day 0

Filgrastim 300 mcg subcutaneously daily

Furosemide (Lasix) 20 mg IV daily for fluid overload

Medroxyprogesterone (Depo-Provera) 150 mg IM if patient is menstruating

Oprelvekin (Neumega) 5 mg subcutaneously daily starting on day 0

Aminocaproic acid (Amicar) 24 gms in 24 hours (4 gms every 4 hours) to start when platelet count is below 30,000.

Epoetin (Procrit) 40,000 units subcutaneously weekly

What should the nurse teach MG about melphalan?

Melphalan can cause severe hypersensitivity reactions with IV doses. It usually occurs within the first 15 minutes of infusion. The nurse should instruct MG to report generalized itching, nausea, chest tightness, crampy abdominal pain, difficulty speaking, anxiety, agitation, sense of impending doom, uneasiness, desire to urinate/defecate, dizziness, and chills. At high doses, melphalan is highly emotogenic. MG will receive both prechemotherapy and around-the-clock antiemetics. MG will be on neutropenic precautions such as avoiding visitors with infections, no stagnant water, fresh flowers, fresh fruit, or fresh vegetables. All of these things may harbor organisms. She may experience mouth sores, so meticulous mouth care is important. She may experience decreased appetite and will be followed by the nutritionist throughout the hospitalization.[6]

The order for melphalan is 280 mg. Is the dose based on ideal or actual body weight?

It is based on actual or ideal body weight, whichever is less. In this case actual body weight is greater.

The physician orders IV fluids of 1 L D51/2 NSS at 25 ml/hr to start 4 hours prior to melphalan infusion and to continue for 6-12 hours postinfusion. The nurse knows that melphalan requires aggressive hydration.

Is this the correct infusion rate for the hydration fluids for MG? What should the nurse do next?

High-dose melphalan can cause renal and liver toxicities, so aggressive hydration is required to flush out the body. The IV rate of 25 ml/hr is not enough for adequate hydration. The rate should be 150 cc/hr if MG can tolerate it. The nurse calls the physician prior to administering the hydration to check the rate since she knows it is too low for this type of protocol.

MG tolerates the melphalan without difficulty. She complains of some intermittent nausea and the nurse gives her the antiemetics that were ordered. MG told the nurse during the intake session that ginger often helped her with nausea and vomiting with her previous chemotherapy. She brought some with her and wants to use it.

What should the nurse tell her?

The nurse explains that MG should wait to use the ginger until the nurse checks with her physician because it may interact with the medications she is receiving.[7]

Twenty-four hours prior to the start of reinfusion, MG is to receive IV fluids of 1 L NSS at 150 cc/hr with 1 amp sodium bicarbonate (NaHCO$_3$). What is the rationale behind this type of hydration?

This is to ensure adequate hydration and protect MG's kidneys. The NaHCO$_3$ helps keep the urine alkaline so that the melphalan will not crystallize in MG's kidneys in an acidic environment. The pH should be above 7. The fluids help to flush the chemotherapy out of her kidneys.[4]

If the urine pH is abnormal what should the nurse do?

If the pH drops below 7, the nurse needs to get an order to administer additional NaHCO$_3$.

What symptoms and side effects might the nurse anticipate that MG may experience during the APBSCT course?

MG will experience myelosuppression, and she might experience stomatitis and venoocclusive disease. Other complications could include catheter-related infections.

Meticulous mouth care and oral assessment every shift is important. Catheter-related care using the proper techniques for dressing changes and catheter care as per hospital policies and procedures can prevent infections. The nurse should assess the insertion site every time she uses the central line. She should monitor vital signs every 4 hours because a temperature could be a sign of a catheter infection. Myelosuppression occurs due to the high doses of chemotherapy used to ablate the bone marrow in preparation of the transplant. Proper hand washing is the best defense in prevention of infection. Monitoring the patient's weight and measuring the abdominal girth can give an indication of venoocclusive disease. This occurs due to the damage to the liver from high-dose chemotherapy and radiation. Patients with venoocclusive disease will have a weight gain and fluid retention and become jaundiced. Therefore, daily weights and an increase in abdominal girth could be early indicators of a problem. Additional measures include monitoring lab results such as liver function tests, assessing vital signs, and strict intake and output recording.[8]

MG is ready for her stem cell reinfusion. She has 12 bags of cells to be infused. The nurse assists MG in getting ready for the reinfusion. She started aggressive hydration with mannitol and $NaHCO_3$ the evening prior to reinfusion. She gets premedicated with acetaminophen (Tylenol), diphenhydramine (Benadryl), dexamethasone, mannitol, and lorazepam. She is placed on a cardiac monitor and a pulse oximeter. Vital signs are taken prior to the beginning of the infusion, prior to each bag, and at the end.

What adverse effects could occur during the stem cell reinfusion?

Adverse effects that may occur during the infusion include nausea, vomiting, abdominal cramping, diarrhea, facial flushing, hypertension, hypotension, bradycardia, tachycardia, other cardiac arrhythmias, tachypnea, dyspnea, cough chest tightness, fever, chills, and hemoglobinurea.[4]

Why do most adverse effects related to stem cell infusion occur?

Most adverse effects occur because of dimethyl sulfoxide (DMSO), the cryoprotectant used for preserving the stem cells. Hydration will keep the kidneys functioning normally and the sodium bicarbonate and mannitol will promote osmotic diuresis. The other premedications are ordered to diminish the reactions to DMSO.[4]

The reinfusion goes well. MG complains of an unusual garlicky taste in her mouth after the reinfusion.

Is this a normal occurrence, and if so, what is its cause? What nursing interventions could be provided for MG related to the garlicky taste?

Yes, this is a normal occurrence during the reinfusion process. Most patients complain of a garlicky taste due to DMSO. To help combat this, most patients drink frequently and suck on hard candy to help get rid of the taste. It will last about

24-48 hours. Family and staff will notice a garlicky odor on the patient's breath, skin, and in her urine.[4]

Fluconazole 100 mg orally daily is ordered starting on the day of reinfusion. Why is this ordered?

It is ordered because immunosuppressed APBSCT patients could be prone to developing fungal infections.[9]

The day after reinfusion MG starts having diarrhea. How can the nurse intervene?

The nurse should notify the physician about the diarrhea. She monitors MG's stool count and intake and output. She obtains stool cultures for *C. difficile* and ova and parasites. She medicates MG with an antidiarrheal as ordered after the cultures are obtained.[9]

On day 3 postinfusion, MG complains of a sore mouth and sore throat. She rates her pain a 5 out of 10 on the pain scale.

What are the nursing interventions?

The nurse continues to offer frequent mouth care—at least 5 times a day—and use of a soft toothbrush. Oral assessment is done every shift. A nutritionist sees MG to alter her diet to softer, high-protein foods that do not irritate her mouth. MG should avoid acidic and spicy foods. The nurse continues to offer MG oxycodone and acetaminophen 5/325 as ordered before meals and as needed. If the pain becomes more severe, she could obtain an order for a low-dose morphine PCA pump.[9]

On day 5 MG spikes a temperature of 101.5°F. What should the nurse do?

MG is approaching her nadir at this point. The nurse notifies the physician because blood cultures will need to be ordered and antibiotics promptly started. She continues to monitor her vital signs q 4 hours or more frequently as indicated.

In addition, strict neutropenic precautions should be followed. Strict hand washing is the most important way to reduce infection.[4]

MG receives the following growth factors: filgrastim, oprelvekin, and epoetin. Her blood count has dropped to the following:

Hemoglobin and hematocrit: 7 g/dL and 22%
WBC: 0.9 millimeter^3 (mm^3)
Platelets: 22,000 platelets per mm^3

Why are these drugs ordered?

Since MG is a Jehovah's Witness and participating in the bloodless medicine program, administering growth factors is a normal part of the treatment to encourage cellular growth. Filgrastim is given to stimulate or boost white blood cell production. It works with the body's natural defense system to help restore the white blood cells. Oprelvekin is a growth factor that stimulates the production of platelets and helps to prevent extremely low platelet counts. Epoetin is given to stimulate red blood cell production.[4,10]

Aminocaproic acid is ordered for MG. Why is this being given?

Aminocaproic acid inhibits fibrinolysis by inhibiting plasminogen activator substances. It prevents clots from breaking down. This is important in preventing MG from bleeding with a low platelet count.[10]

What other nursing measures can be implemented for MG?

The nurse should make sure MG is on thrombocytopenic precautions. She should instruct her to avoid invasive procedures such as IM injections or blood draws, straining with bowel movements, or shaving with a straight razor. Institute safety measures to prevent injury, such as nightlights, walking to the bathroom with a staff member at night, using a soft toothbrush, and wearing slippers with treads on the soles to prevent slipping.[11]

If MG was of childbearing age, she would be given medroxyprogesterone. Why would this medication be used?

It would be used to halt her menstrual cycle so that blood loss would be minimized.[6]

MG's hemoglobin and hematocrit start rising on day 14. Her WBC starts rising on day 16 and her platelet count recovers on the 21st day.[4]

Is this a normal occurrence?

Yes, this is about the time that blood counts show recovery and engraftment occurs.

MG continues to do well and recovers without any further difficulties. She returns home 6 weeks after the start of the transplant. She is still in remission at 1 year and is being followed by her local oncologist. She states she has gone back to her usual activities and is enjoying her family.

REFERENCES

1. The Center for Bloodless Medicine and Surgery at Pennsylvania Hospital. Non-blood management techniques. Available at: http://pennhealth.com/bloodless/management.htm#diet. Accessed August 1, 2006.

2. Itano JK. Coping: cultural issues. In: Itano JK, Toka KN, eds. *Core Curriculum for Oncology Nursing.* 4th ed. St Louis, MO: Elsevier Saunders; 2005:59-77.

3. Pokorny KS. Stem cell collection. In: Ezzone S, ed. *Hematopoietic Stem Cell Transplantation: A Manual for Nursing Practice.* Pittsburgh, PA: Oncology Nursing Press; 2004:23-42.

4. Walker-McAdams F, Reilly-Burgunder M. Transplant course. In: Ezzone S, ed. *Hematopoietic Stem Cell Transplantation: A Manual for Nursing Practice.* Pittsburgh, PA: Oncology Nursing Press; 2004:43-59.

5. Cyracom International Transparent Language Services. Available at: www.cyracom.com. Accessed November 21, 2005.

6. Wilkes GM, Barton-Burke M. *2005 Oncology Drug Handbook.* Sudbury, MA: Jones and Bartlett; 2005:209-212, 262-263.

7. Ross PJ. Complementary and alternative medicines. In: Itano KN, Toka K, eds. *Core Curriculum for Oncology Nursing.* 4th ed. Philadelphia, PA: Elsevier Saunders Company; 2005:828-836.

8. Buschel PC, Leum E, Randolph SR. Nursing care of the blood cell transplant patient. *Semin Oncol Nurs.* 1997;113(3):172-183.

9. Wilkle-Shapiro T. Nursing implications of hematopoietic stem cell transplantation In: Itano JK, Taoka KN, eds. *Core Curriculum for Oncology Nursing.* 4th ed. St Louis, MO: Elsevier Saunders; 2005:808-826.

10. Ballen KK, Becker PS, Yeap BY, Matthews B, Henry DH, Ford PA. Autologous stem-cell transplantation can be performed safely without the use of blood-product support. *J Clin Oncol.* 2004;22(20):4087-4094.

11. Camp-Sorrell D. Myelosuppression. In: Itano JK, Taoka KN, eds. *Core Curriculum for Oncology Nursing.* 4th ed. St. Louis, MO: Elsevier Saunders; 2005:264-267.

Leukemia and Thrombocytopenia Case Study

SG is a 28-year-old female recently diagnosed with acute myelogenous leukemia (AML). She was diagnosed during the third trimester of her pregnancy when she presented with fatigue, an elevated white blood cell count, and diffuse adenopathy. SG delivered a healthy baby boy at 38 weeks via cesarean section. She is admitted to the oncology unit for her first cycle of induction therapy 5 days after delivery. Lab values include CBC, hemoglobin 12 g/dl, hematocrit 36%, platelets 300,000, WBC 400,000 with 60% blast cells, BUN 0.9 mg/dl, and creatine 1.0 mg/dl. Liver function tests are within normal limits. SG is married and has a supportive family and network of friends. SG weighs 132 lbs and is 5 feet 4 inches tall. Her physician orders the following induction chemotherapy regimen:

Idarubicin (Idamycin) 6 mg/m2/day IV days 1-5
Cytarabine (Ara-C) 2000 mg/m2/dose IV every 12 hours days 1-5 for a total of 10 doses
Etoposide (VP-16) 100 mg/day IV days 1-5
Antiemetics:
Ondansetron (Zofran) 8 mg IV every 12 hours

Dexamethasone (Decadron) 20 mg IV once a day

Antiemetics are to be continued for 24 hours after chemotherapy.

What is induction therapy?

Induction is the initial treatment with high-dose chemotherapy agents given with the goal of eradicating the leukemia cells and putting the patient into complete remission. More treatment then follows to achieve long-term, disease-free survival. Options include consolidation therapy, intensification therapy, maintenance therapy, and bone marrow transplant. Consolidation therapy consists of 2 or 3 more cycles of the same chemotherapy used in induction therapy given after remission occurs. Intensification therapy is high-dose chemotherapy given immediately after or after several months of induction therapy. The same chemotherapy used for induction but at higher doses or chemotherapy drugs thought to be cross-resistant with the initial drugs may be used. Maintenance therapy consists of lower doses of the same drugs used for induction therapy or other drugs given monthly for a long period of time. It is not currently being done in patients with AML. Bone marrow or peripheral stem cell transplant is done with allogeneic or matched unrelated donors. This process has a long-term, disease-free survival rate of 45%-65%. Autologous (the patient's own) bone marrow or peripheral blood stem cell transplant is controversial at this time. A third type of transplant called nonmyeloablative transplant is now being done for patients who are elderly or have risk factors that make them ineligible for myeloablative transplant. The patient receives less toxic chemotherapy. Graft-versus-host-disease with graft-versus-tumor effect is intended to achieve long-term, disease-free survival.[1]

What should the nurse teach SG about her disease and her chemotherapy regimen?

He explains that leukemia is a cancer of the hematopoietic and lymphatic systems most frequently involving white blood cells. Excessive malignant cells crowd out the bone marrow, which impedes normal hematopoietic functioning.[2] AML and chronic lymphocytic leukemia are the most common forms of leukemia in adults.[1] Leukemia is classified based on the predominant cell line affected and maturation reached. Myeloid stem cells differentiate into hematopoietic stem cells including red blood cells, white blood cells, and platelets. The goal of giving induction chemotherapy is to kill the malignant cells in the bone marrow, which allows for new normal cells to grow, putting the patient into remission. The nurse begins the teaching session with discussing the side effects of cytarabine with SG. These include myelosuppression consisting of anemia, neutropenia, and thrombocytopenia, cerebellar toxicity (high dose), possible renal or liver damage, nausea and vomiting, mucositis, photophobia and conjunctivitis, and neurotoxicity. He then discusses the side effects of idarubicin. These also include myelosuppression, nausea and vomiting, stomatitis, and possible liver toxicity. In addition, SG may experience cardiac toxicity in the form of congestive heart failure (CHF) if large, cumulative doses are given. A multi-gated acquisition (MUGA) scan should be done prior to administering idarubicin. Other side effects include anorexia, diarrhea, alopecia, skin changes, and impaired fertility.[3] Next he discusses the side effects of etoposide, which also include nausea, vomiting, anorexia, and alopecia. Orthostatic hypotension is specific to etoposide. The nurse explains to SG that he will be taking blood pressure preinfusion and postinfusion.[3] To reinforce verbal teaching, he gives SG written materials that include drug sheets and information about neutropenia, thrombocytopenia, nausea and vomiting, and signs and symptoms to report. Prior to discharge, SG needs phone contact numbers and information about follow-up appointments. The nurse makes sure that SG has retained the important need-to-know information.[3-4] The clinical signs and symptoms of leukemia are outlined in **Table 22.1**.

As the nurse reviews the chemotherapy orders for SG, he realizes that there are orders missing. What is his next step? What orders are missing?

He asks the physician to order IV hydration for SG. Aggressive hydration is important in newly diagnosed patients with AML to prevent tumor lysis syndrome. He needs to question the physician about ordering allopurinol (Zyloprim) to help lower serum and urinary uric acid levels caused by the breakdown of tumor

Table 22.1   **Manifestations of Leukemia**

Etiology	Manifestation
Granulocytopenia	Fever
	Abdominal pain
	Respiratory infection
	Perirectal abscess
	Adenopathy
	Mucositis
Thrombocytopenia	Purpura, petechiae, ecchymoses
	Bleeding gums
	Epistaxis
	Retinal hemorrhage
	Intracranial bleeding
Anemia	Fatigue or malaise
	Pallor
	Dyspnea
Leukemia infiltrates	Pain or swelling in bones and joints
	Hepatomegaly
	Splenomegaly

Source: From Wuijcik D. Leukemia. In: Yarbro CH, Frogge MH, Goodman M, eds. *Cancer nursing: principles and practice.* 6th ed. Sudbury, MA: Jones and Bartlett; 2005:1248, Manifestations of Leukemia.

cells.[3] The last thing he would ask the physician to order is corticosteroid eye drops since cytarabine causes photophobia and conjunctivitis.[3]

The physician agrees with the nurse and orders the following:

1 L 0.9 NSS IV at 150 cc/hr
Allopurinol 300 mg po bid
Dexamethasone (Maxitrol) eye drops 2 gtts both eyes bid

What is tumor lysis syndrome?

Tumor lysis syndrome is a preventable oncologic emergency. It occurs when there is a rapid release of intracellular material in the blood due to tumor cells dying rapidly. Since SG has a high WBC count due to AML, she is at high risk for this condition. Symptoms include hyperkalemia, hypocalcemia, hyperphosphatemia, hyperuricemia, oliguria, acute renal failure, tetany, cardiac arrhythmias, and cardiopulmonary arrest. The best treatment is aggressive IV hydration to keep urine output at 150 ml or more an hour and allopurinol to decrease uric acid level and prevent hyperuricemia, and alkalinization of urine with sodium bicarbonate. The nurse should monitor intake and output closely. He should monitor lab values closely as electrolyte imbalances need to be corrected. In rare instances, hemodialysis may be necessary for patients who do not respond or for those who develop renal insufficiency.[5-6]

What nursing interventions should the nurse include in his plan of care?

He is concerned with how SG is coping with her diagnosis of AML as well as how she is coping with her new son and husband since the first weeks after birth are the most important in developing a maternal infant bond. He needs to be concerned about SG's husband and how he is coping with his new role and what adjustments he will have to make while SG is in treatment. The nurse offers SG and her family information on many of the supportive services that are available, such as social work, pastoral care, and psychological services. He makes SG aware of the available support groups and gives her the American Cancer Society and Leukemia and Lymphoma Society contact information. Another consideration could be to get assistance from the maternity department to assist SG and her husband in learning about newborn care. He wants to allow SG and her husband as much time with their baby as possible to promote bonding and development of the family unit. He could suggest that SG elicit help from her large group of family and friends to help with child care and routine household functions.

Another area of concern is management of side effects from SG's chemotherapy regimen. The nurse needs to monitor her blood counts, liver, and renal function tests on a daily basis. Nursing interventions would include monitoring of vital signs every 4 hours, including a neurological assessment. When cerebellar toxicity from cytarabine develops, it is usually 5 days after treatment and can last for up to 1 week. CNS toxicities are usually mild and reversible. Neurology checks should be done at least once a shift. The nurse monitors urine pH on SG's urine to keep the pH above 7. Strict intake and output is a must.[3]

SG had a cesarean section and would be at risk for infection and poor wound healing due to her receiving chemotherapy and having an abdominal wound post-delivery. The nurse assesses the healing process of SG's abdominal wound every 8 hours.

SG receives her induction regimen without difficulty. Four days after chemotherapy, SG complains of soreness at her C-section site. Upon assessment, her incision is red and has some malodorous drainage. The blood counts for SG are hemoglobin 9 g/dl, hematocrit 33%, WBC 3.0, and platelets 60,000. SG also starts running a low-grade fever.

What is happening to SG and what are the nursing actions?

It appears that SG has developed a wound infection and is becoming myelosuppressed. She has a low-grade fever, a draining wound, and is close to her nadir period when her blood cell counts are at their lowest. The nurse notifies her physician as well as her obstetrician and continues to monitor her vital signs every 4 hours. SG will be put on a broad-spectrum antibiotic and needs wound care to her C-section site. In addition, the physician may order cultures of the drainage from her wound. SG's nurse keeps her informed about what is happening and provides support.

The physician orders a cefepime (Maxipeme) antibiotic 2 grams IV every 8 hours times 7 days or until neutrophil recovery.

Why is this ordered for SG?

Cefepime (Maxipeme) is a broad-spectrum antibiotic used to treat infections as well as empiric therapy for febrile neutropenia.[3]

On day 10 postchemotherapy, SG has a temperature of 101.5°F. She is complaining of fatigue and says her gums are bleeding when she brushes her teeth and has small red dots the size of a pencil point on her upper and lower extremities.

Her labs are as follows: Her Hgb and Hct are 8.0g/dl and 30%, her WBC 2.0, her segs 50%, bands 7%, and platelets 20,000/mm². Her liver and renal lab values are within normal limits.

Calculate SG's absolute neutrophil count (ANC). If she is neutropenic, what nursing interventions should be implemented?

$$\text{ANC} = 50\% \text{ segs} + 7\% \text{ bands} \times 1000 = (0.5 + 0.07) \times 1000$$
$$\text{ANC} = 570$$

SG is neutropenic and at risk for infection. (See Chapter 12 for more information about neutropenia.) Her nurse implements neutropenic precautions such as careful hand washing, which he should be doing with every patient contact. SG should not have any visitors who may be sick. The nadir that occurs with SG's chemotherapy usually occurs between days 7 and 10 with recovery of blood counts between days 14 and 21. Since SG is febrile and it is her nadir period, she may be becoming septic. Immediate action is needed. Please see the neutropenic case study in Chapter 12 for further details about care of the neutropenic patient.

What else about SG's blood counts stands out, and what should her nurse add to his plan of care as a result?

SG has a low platelet count. A normal platelet count is 150,000 to 400,000/mm³. Since SG has a count of 20,000, she is considered thrombocytopenic. There is a decrease in the number of platelets being produced and the destruction of mature platelet cells with chemotherapy-related thrombocytopenia. Circulating platelets have a lifespan of 8-10 days. Platelet count usually decreases 7-14 days after chemotherapy and occurs after WBCs drop. Normal platelet recovery occurs in 2-6 weeks. When the platelet level falls below 20,000/mm^3, a patient is considered at major risk for spontaneous bleeding. Bed rest should be maintained when the platelet count falls below 10,000/mm^3 because the patient is at risk for spontaneous CNS, GI, or respiratory bleeding. As far as assessment data that may indicate thrombocytopenia, SG has petechiae on her upper and lower extremities and she is experiencing increased bleeding and bruising. Other assessment data includes checking all excreta for blood, monitoring SG for change in mental status such as restlessness, headache, change in level of consciousness, seizures, pupil changes, and ataxia. CNS changes could indicate spontaneous bleeding.

Her nurse will most likely administer platelets when her platelet count falls below 10,000-20,000/mm^3. He should teach SG about bleeding precautions and begin interventions that would minimize bleeding. These interventions include avoiding invasive procedures such as SQ or IM injections, rectal temperatures, bladder catheterization, and nasogastric tubes. The nurse should hold venipuncture sites for at least 5 minutes. He should provide a safe environment for SG and teach her to avoid sharp objects such as straight razors. He should encourage her to wear shoes or slippers when ambulating and use a soft toothbrush when brushing her teeth. He should start SG on a bowel regimen to avoid constipation. A patient at home with low platelets would be encouraged to avoid heavy physical activity. SG may receive a platelet growth factor such as oprelvekin (Neumega).[7] The National Cancer Institute Common Toxicity Criteria grading system helps nurses determine the severity of thrombocytopenia (**Table 22.2**).

SG is discharged on day 16 with stable vital signs. Her counts are returning to normal and she is discharged to follow up with her oncologist for further treatment.

The nurse sees SG's physician at a case conference 2 weeks later where SG's case is being presented. He learns that SG and her family are doing quite well. She is preparing to come in to the hospital next week for her consolidation regimen. Her physician states that he is going to add pegfilgrastim (Neulasta) to her treatment with her next admission.

Table 22.2   National Cancer Institute Common Toxicity Criteria: Platelets

			Grade		
Toxicity	0	1	2	3	4
Platelets	WNL	< LLN–< 75.0 × 10⁹/L	≥ 50.0–< 75.0 × 10⁹/L	≥ 10.0–< 50.0 × 10⁹/L	< 10.0 × 10⁹/L
		< LLN–75,000/mm³	≥ 50,000–< 75,000/mm³	≥ 10,000–< 50,000/mm³	< 10,000/mm³

Source: Wilkes GM, Barton-Burke M. *2005 Oncology Nursing Drug Handbook.* Sudbury, MA: Jones and Bartlett, 2005:989.

What is pegfilgrastim and why is it ordered for SG along with her next treatment?

Pegfilgrastim is a colony-stimulating growth factor that stimulates the growth of WBCs. It decreases the incidence of febrile neutropenia in patients who are receiving chemotherapy and at risk for severe febrile neutropenia. It helps keep chemotherapy administration on schedule. It is given subcutaneously in a dosage of 6 mg. It is given once per chemotherapy cycle on the day after treatment, which means less travel to the oncologist's office for the patient and family. The main side effect that patients will experience is bone pain, which can be relieved with a nonsteroidal anti-inflammatory agent.[3-4]

REFERENCES

1. Moran MJ, Ezzone S. Nursing care of the client with leukemia. In: Itano JK, Taoka KN, eds. *Core Curriculum for Oncology Nursing.* 4th ed. St. Louis, MO: Elsevier Saunders; 2005:676-687.

2. Goodman M, Hayden B. Chemotherapy: Principles of administration. In: Yarbro CH, Frogge MG, Goodman M, Groenwald SL, eds. *Cancer Nursing Principles and Practice.* 6th ed. Sudbury, MA: Jones and Bartlett; 2005:1336-1339.

3. Wilkes GM, Barton-Burke M. *2005 Oncology Drug Handbook.* Sudbury, MA: Jones and Bartlett; 2005:156-160, 184-186, 356-359, 383-386, 757-758.

4. Chu E, Devita V. *Cancer Chemotherapy Drug Manual*. Sudbury, MA: Jones and Bartlett, 2005:107-111,291-293.

5. Gobel BH. Metabolic emergencies. In: Itano JK, Taoka KN, eds. *Core Curriculum for Oncology Nursing*. 4th ed. St. Louis, MO: Elsevier Saunders; 2005:395-400.

6. Lynch MP. *Essentials of Oncology Care*. New York: Professional Publishing Group; 2005:172.

7. Camp-Sorrell D. Myelosuppression. In: Itano JK, Taoka KN, eds. *Core Curriculum for Oncology Nursing*. 4th ed. St. Louis, MO: Elsevier Saunders; 2005:264-267.

23

Venous Access Device Case Study

MP is a 40-year-old female with newly diagnosed breast cancer. She will be receiving 4 cycles of doxorubicin (Adriamycin) and cyclophosphamide (Cytoxan) followed by 4 cycles of paclitaxel (Taxol). MP's oncologist tells her that treatment will begin as soon as an implanted port is placed.

MP asks for more information about the implanted port including the risks and benefits. She is very interested in what the procedure will be like and what to expect after it is placed.

What should the nurse tell her?

An implanted port (**Figure 23.1**) will prevent wear and tear on MP's veins and potentially spare her pain and anxiety related to multiple IV sticks. The implanted port is made of 2 parts: a portal body or septum and the catheter itself. It can be single or double lumen. Ideally, the implanted port is placed on the chest wall just under the collarbone but over a rib for stability. The procedure takes place in the operating room or interventional radiology. It can be placed under local anesthesia with sedation or general anesthesia. Usually it is done under fluoroscopy so that catheter tip placement can be easily confirmed. Otherwise it is

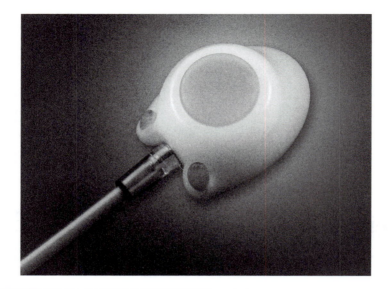

Figure 23.1 **Bard implanted port.**
Source: Used with permission from Bard Access Systems.

confirmed by chest X-ray. The most common veins selected for implanted ports placed on the chest are the subclavian and internal and external jugular. The catheter portion is placed using a cut down or through the skin. MP will have a small insertion site incision that is closed with steri-strips. Next the portal septum is housed in a pocket created under the skin and sutured in place. The pocket area will have an incision as well but not directly over the portal septum to maintain integrity of the incision. If the port will be used right away, a noncoring Huber needle will be left in place because postoperative swelling could make access difficult. The procedure does have risks associated with it, including infection and bleeding.[1]

MP asks if any other options are available to her. How might the nurse respond?

Some patients receive their chemotherapy through a peripheral line. This gets increasingly more difficult as time goes on and an acceptable vein is difficult to find. Not readily finding a vein or being stuck several times can create unnecessary anxiety. Doxorubicin is a vesicant and could cause tissue necrosis if an extravasation does occur. An implanted port is ideal because it is placed under the skin and requires no care except for a monthly flush unless it is accessed. Therefore, there is no dressing change or flushing that MP would have to do at home. This is ideal for patients who have difficulty caring for an external line. A PICC line is a peripherally inserted central catheter. It can be placed under sterile conditions in many different locations such as the bedside or at home, but like all central venous access devices (VADs), it requires confirmation that catheter tip placement is in the superior vena cava above the right atrium. The PICC requires twice-daily flushes and weekly cap and dressing changes. In addition, there is an external catheter in the arm that is noticeable. Peripherally placed ports work well for patients who have open wounds, tumor involvement, or other chest pathology. A peripherally placed port is found above or below the antecubital fossa.[1]

MP has her implanted port placed in the hospital interventional radiology department. The procedure is uneventful. She is discharged to home. What discharge teaching should MP receive?

MP is instructed to leave a dressing on both the insertion and exit sites for 3 days, and then leave the incisions open to air. She is instructed to report any fever or unusual bleeding since the complications of this procedure could be infection and bleeding. She is given a prescription for oxycodone with acetaminophen (Percocet) for pain and is instructed to take 2 tablets every 4 hours as needed for pain. She is informed that the pain should lessen each day over the course of 3 days and will most likely notice minimal pain after those 3 days.

What 2 factors are necessary to confirm before using the port for the first time?

The nurse should confirm that the catheter tip is placed in the superior vena cava and she should check for the presence of brisk blood return.[1-2]

MP comes in to the clinic for her first cycle of chemotherapy. The nurse accesses her port to draw blood and leaves it accessed for chemotherapy. Describe her technique.

MP's nurse needs to access the port using a sterile technique. First she washes her hands and gathers supplies. She will need sterile gloves, a 2% chlorahexadine prep (Chloraprep) (if the chlorahexadine prep is unavailable, she'll need 3 each of povidone-iodine and alcohol swabs), a noncoring Huber needle, usually three fourths to 1 inch, and a transparent dressing. Before she puts her gloves on, she gently palpates the center of the portal septum. After putting her gloves on, she uses the 2% chlorahexadine gluconate to clean the area, making concentric circles starting in the center of the port septum and being careful not to go over the same area twice. Then she holds the noncoring needle with the dominant hand and uses the nondominant hand (thumb and forefinger) to stabilize the septum. She pushes the noncoring needle through the skin and diaphragm and stops when she feels the bottom of the implanted port. She places a transparent dressing over the site so that she can easily visualize the needle.[1]

MP uneventfully receives 3 cycles of chemotherapy. When she returns for her fourth cycle, the nurse is unable to obtain a blood return from the implanted port. She is easily able to instill the saline flush (alternatively, she could have used heparin). MP appears anxious and asks the nurse to draw her blood peripherally and start the chemotherapy.

What is occurring? What can the nurse do next?

MP is experiencing a partial venous access device occlusion. It is most likely a fibrin sheath based on the nurse's ability to infuse the saline flush and her inability to obtain a blood return.[1] She still needs to troubleshoot the situation.

She flushes the catheter gently, using the push-pull method, and then repositions the patient. She asks MP to cough. If there is still no blood, she explains that this is a common occurrence and a delay in treatment is necessary. She reassures MP that the situation is resolvable.[2]

Why is it important to intervene when there is no blood return from a venous access device?

A blood return helps confirm correct placement of the port and the needle used to access it. If placement is confirmed, absence of blood return could indicate the presence of catheter occlusion. If the occlusion is complete, the patient is at risk for developing catheter rupture if too much force is used when attempting to flush the line or the syringe is smaller than 10 ml and too much pressure is upon the catheter. This situation is especially dangerous if a vesicant extravasates because there could be necrotic damage to the tissue surrounding the port. The patient is at risk for infection from either a total or partial occlusion. Retrograde extravasation can occur.[1]

Describe possible causes of either partial or total venous access device occlusion.

There are 5 common causes of venous access device occlusion. The first is when blood and fibrin collects within the lumen of the catheter. This type is known as an intraluminal occlusion. The second type of occlusion is when a fibrin tail or sheath adheres to the tip of the catheter and the outside surface. This tail or sheath acts as a one-way valve allowing fluids to be infused but no blood to be withdrawn. This is the type of occlusion seen in our case study. The third type of occlusion occurs when incompatible solutions are infused or inadequate flushing occurs, causing a drug crystallization to occlude the catheter. The fourth type of occlusion is known as mural thrombosis. This occurs when the fibrin from the catheter surface binds with fibrin from a vessel wall injury and a thrombus is formed. The fifth type of occlusion is simply from the port needle not being in the proper position.[1]

Since the nurse has determined that MP has a fibrin sheath based on the ability to infuse fluids and inability to withdraw blood from the catheter, how could she treat this type of occlusion?

She can obtain an order for and then instill t-PA (Alteplace) 2 mg mixed in 2 ml sterile water. She can use a 10 ml syringe to decrease pressure on the catheter. She should wait from 30 minutes to 2 hours and aspirate and then remove the 2 ml of t-PA and about 5 cc of blood since it may contain the blood or fibrin in it. She may repeat the procedure once if she is unsuccessful. The device should be removed if the situation is not resolved. A dye study done in the radiology department can be useful to visualize the tip of the catheter and to confirm catheter placement and to rule out catheter malfunction or migration.[2] Urokinase is no longer used for VAD occlusion. Reteplase (Retavase) and other recombinant forms of t-PA are being studied for effectiveness in VAD occlusion and are currently approved for myocardial infarction only.[1]

How does t-PA work?

It activates plasminogen to the active enzyme plasmin and degrades clots and fibrin buildup.

Why could MP develop a catheter-related infection if the fibrin sheath is not resolved?

The fibrin sheath forms a matrix for bacteria to adhere onto. The combination of the bacteria and the fibrin produce an extracellular slime that allows the bacteria to be undetected by antibodies and to proliferate.[1]

What are the risk factors for developing venous access device occlusion?

Risk factors for developing VAD occlusion include the type of malignancy the patient has (for example, lung cancer is associated with increased clotting), the patient's own physiologic clotting response, inadequate routine flushing (particularly after withdrawing blood from the catheter), size and composition of the catheter itself, irritating materials (some materials are more irritating to the vein), a catheter tip located in the lower third of the superior vena cava, and infusion of incompatible solutions causing drug crystallization.[1]

How can venous access device occlusions be prevented?

The most important thing one can do to prevent VAD occlusion is to flush adequately after using the catheter or drawing blood. The nurse should be especially careful when drawing blood. She should always flush with 20 ml saline in that situation. Warfarin (Coumadin) at a low dose of 1 mg a day could decrease the possibility of developing an occlusion but potentially could increase the risk of bleeding.[1]

REFERENCES

1. Camp-Sorrell D, ed. *Access Device Guidelines: Recommendations for Nursing Practice and Education.* 2nd ed. Pittsburgh, PA: Oncology Nursing Society; 2004:3-48.

2. Polovich M, White JM, Kelleher LO, eds. *Chemotherapy and Biotherapy Guidelines and Recommendations for Practice.* 2nd ed. Pittsburgh, PA: Oncology Nursing Society; 2005:74-75.

Index